CSBS DP™ Manual

Communication
and Symbolic
Behavior Scales
Developmental Profile
First Normed Edition

CSBS DP™ Manual

Communication and Symbolic Behavior Scales Developmental Profile™

First Normed Edition

Amy M. Wetherby, Ph.D., CCC-SLP
Florida State University
Tallahassee, Florida

Barry M. Prizant, Ph.D., CCC-SLP
Childhood Communication Services
Cranston, Rhode Island

Paul H. Brookes Publishing Co.

Baltimore • London • Sydney

·P A U L·H·
BROOKES
PUBLISHING CO.®

Paul H. Brookes Publishing Co.
Post Office Box 10624
Baltimore, Maryland 21285-0624

www.brookespublishing.com

Typeset by Type Shoppe II Productions, Ltd., Chestertown, Maryland.
Manufactured in the United States of America by
Versa Press, Inc., East Peoria, Illinois.

Case studies and real names are used by permission.

The following CSBS DP forms can be purchased separately:

- *CSBS DP Forms, First Normed Edition:* package includes 25 Infant-Toddler Checklists, 25 Caregiver Questionnaires, 25 Behavior Sample: Scoring Worksheets, 25 Caregiver Perception Rating forms, 25 Infant-Toddler Checklist: Screening Reports, and 1 Outline of Sampling Procedures and Instructions card.
- *CSBS DP Caregiver Questionnaire:* package of 50

To order, contact Paul H. Brookes Publishing Co., Post Office Box 10624, Baltimore, Maryland 21285-0624 (1-800-638-3775; 410-337-9580; http://www.brookespublishing.com/csbsdp)

See the back of this manual for more information about the CSBS DP product line. All products are available from Paul H. Brookes Publishing Co.

Library of Congress Cataloging-in-Publication Data

Wetherby, Amy M.
Communication and symbolic behavior scales: developmental profile/Amy M. Wetherby and Barry M. Prizant.—1st normed ed.
p. cm.
Includes bibliographical references and index.
ISBN 1-55766-556-7
1. Communication and Symbolic Behavior Scales Developmental Profile. 2. Infants—Psychological testing. I. Prizant, Barry M. (Barry Mitchell) II. Title.

BF719.65.C65 W48 2002
155.4'36'0287—dc21 2002016092

British Library Cataloguing in Publication data are available from the British Library.

CONTENTS

ABOUT THE AUTHORS

Amy M. Wetherby, Ph.D., CCC-SLP, Laurel Schendel Professor of Communication Disorders, Department of Communication Disorders, Florida State University, Tallahassee, FL 32306

Dr. Wetherby received her doctorate from the University of California, San Francisco/Santa Barbara in 1982. She has more than 20 years of clinical experience in the design and implementation of communication programs for children with autism and severe communication impairments and is a Fellow of the American Speech-Language-Hearing Association. Dr. Wetherby's research has focused on communicative and cognitive-social aspects of language problems in children with autism and on the early identification of children with communication impairments. She has published extensively on these topics and presents regularly at national conventions. She is a co-author of the *Communication and Symbolic Behavior Scales* (with Barry M. Prizant; Paul H. Brookes Publishing Co., 1993) and *Autism Spectrum Disorders: A Transactional Developmental Perspective* (co-edited with Barry M. Prizant; Paul H. Brookes Publishing Co., 2000).

Dr. Wetherby is the Project Director of the FIRST WORDS Project http://firstwords.fsu.edu) funded by a U.S. Department of Education Field-Initiated Research Grant on improving early identification of young children at risk for language and reading difficulties and a Model Demonstration Grant on early identification of communication disorders in infants and toddlers. She is also the Project Co-Director (with Juliann Woods) of the Early Social Interaction Project funded by a U.S. Department of Education Model Demonstration Grant on the effectiveness of a comprehensive early intervention program for very young children with autism spectrum disorders. Dr. Wetherby served on the National Academy of Sciences Committee for Educational Interventions for Children with Autism and is the Executive Director of the Florida State University Center for Autism and Related Disabilities.

Barry M. Prizant, Ph.D., CCC-SLP, Adjunct Professor, Center for Human Development, Brown University, Providence, RI; Director, Childhood Communication Services, 2024 Broad Street, Cranston, RI 02905

Dr. Prizant has more than 25 years of experience as a clinical scholar, researcher, and consultant to young children with autism spectrum disorders (ASD) and other childhood disabilities and their families. He is Director of Childhood Communication Services, an Adjunct Professor in the Center for Human Development at Brown University, and a Fellow of the American Speech-Language-Hearing Association. Formerly, he was an Associate Professor of Psychiatry in the Brown University Program in Medicine; Director of the Communication Disorders Department at Bradley Hospital in Providence, Rhode Island; and an Advanced Postdoctoral Fellow in Early Intervention at the University of North Carolina at Chapel Hill. He has developed and co-directed family-centered programs for newly diagnosed toddlers with ASD and their families in hospital and university clinic settings.

Dr. Prizant is author or co-author of more than 90 articles and chapters, co-editor (with Amy Wetherby) of *Autism Spectrum Disorders: A Transactional Developmental Perspective* (Paul H. Brookes Publishing Co., 2000), and an editorial consultant for five professional journals in the areas of autism spectrum disorders and communication/language development and disorders. He has presented seminars and keynote addresses at conferences throughout North America, Europe, the Middle East, and the Far East. He also is an advisory board member of the Interdisciplinary Council on Developmental and Learning Disorders (Dr. Stanley Greenspan, Chair) and First Signs, Inc., an organization working to improve early diagnosis and referral. Dr. Prizant's current research and clinical interests include relationships between communication and social and emotional development, and identification and family-centered treatment of infants, toddlers, and young children who have or are at risk for social-communication difficulties, including ASD.

To Tom Hutchinson and Bill Hammack
for their belief in and support of the
Communication and Symbolic Behavior Scales
and for their perseverance and encouragement
throughout the development of the CSBS DP

OVERVIEW 1

The Communication and Symbolic Behavior Scales Developmental Profile™ (CSBS DP_{TM}) is a standardized tool designed to evaluate communication and symbolic abilities of children whose functional communication age is between 6 months and 2 years. It may also be used with preschool children whose chronological age is up to 5–6 years if their developmental level of functioning is younger than 24 months. The purpose of the CSBS DP is threefold:

1. For screening to identify children at risk for developmental delay or disability who need a developmental evaluation
2. For evaluation to determine if a child has delays in social communication, expressive speech/language, and symbolic functioning
3. For evaluation to document changes in social communication, expressive speech/language, and symbolic functioning over time

Because of its brevity, the CSBS DP should not be used alone as the basis for decision making in program planning. It should be used as a guide to indicate areas that need further assessment or as an evaluation tool to monitor change. The Communication and Symbolic Behavior Scales™ ($CSBS_{TM}$), Normed Edition (Wetherby & Prizant, 1993), is a more in-depth tool and is designed for decision making in program planning.

TWO-STEP SCREENING AND EVALUATION PROCESS

The CSBS DP consists of three components:

1. One-page CSBS DP Infant-Toddler Checklist for screening
2. Four-page CSBS DP Caregiver Questionnaire for follow-up evaluation
3. Thirty-minute CSBS DP Behavior Sample for a face-to-face evaluation of the child

The Infant-Toddler Checklist, Caregiver Questionnaire, and all forms required for scoring them, as well as for scoring the Behavior Sample, are included in the test kit.

The CSBS DP is a two-step process—the first step is screening with the CSBS DP Infant-Toddler Checklist, and, if needed, the second step is evaluating with the CSBS DP Caregiver Questionnaire and CSBS DP Behavior Sample, as diagramed in Figure 1.1.

What Does the CSBS DP Measure?

The CSBS DP screens and evaluates a child's social communication, expressive speech/language, and symbolic abilities based on parent report and face-to-face

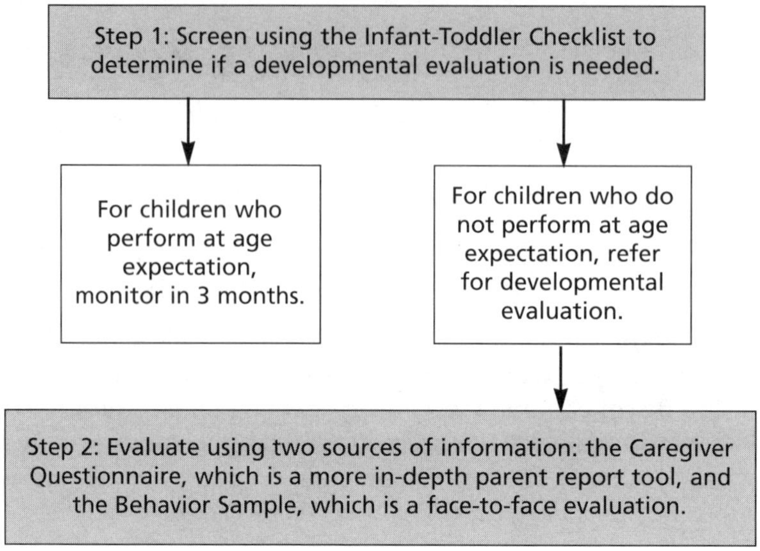

Figure 1.1. CSBS DP two-step process.

evaluation. Each of the three components measures seven cluster areas that are organized into three composites.

Social Composite

- Emotion and Eye Gaze
- Communication
- Gestures

Speech Composite

- Sounds
- Words

Symbolic Composite

- Understanding
- Object Use

HOW IS THE CSBS DP ADMINISTERED?

The CSBS DP Infant-Toddler Checklist and the CSBS DP Caregiver Questionnaire provide important information about a child's abilities based on caregiver report. The CSBS DP Behavior Sample is a face-to-face evaluation for professionals that uses a standard but flexible format for sampling behavior from young children. The sampling procedures consist of the following strategies designed to encourage spontaneous behavior. The strategies range in degree of structure provided by the adults.

- Communicative temptations, which are situations designed to entice a child to communicate
- Book sharing

- Symbolic play, using a feeding set to encourage pretending with objects
- Language comprehension probes
- Constructive play, using blocks to encourage stacking

Materials used during the CSBS DP Behavior Sample include action-based toys to entice spontaneous communication, books designed for young children, and play materials that evaluate how a child uses and plays with objects symbolically and constructively. Materials are presented in a designated sequence with minimal intrusion or direction. The child's caregiver is present and is instructed to respond naturally but not direct the child's behavior in order to encourage spontaneous communication and play. The caregiver is involved in the CSBS DP in three ways:

1. As a reporter and describer, by completing the CSBS DP Infant-Toddler Checklist and Caregiver Questionnaire
2. As a participant, by being present and interacting with the child during the CSBS DP Behavior Sample
3. As a validator, by completing the CSBS DP Behavior Sample: Caregiver Perception Rating to indicate how typical the child's behavior was during the sample

Who Can Administer the CSBS DP?

The CSBS DP can be administered by a certified speech-language pathologist, early interventionist, psychologist, or other professional trained to evaluate developmentally young children.

How Long Does it Take to Administer and Score?

The CSBS DP Infant-Toddler Checklist can be completed by a parent or caregiver in about 5–10 minutes. The CSBS DP Caregiver Questionnaire can be completed by a parent or caregiver in about 20 minutes and can be mailed ahead or given to the caregiver at the evaluation. The CSBS DP Behavior Sample takes about 30 minutes to complete, including a brief warm-up period in which both the child and caregiver should participate. The Behavior Sample can be scored during the sample by a trained evaluator. It may also be videotaped to document the child's performance and to enable the evaluator to score it later or to check the scoring. Video recording is not necessary unless the evaluator or parent wants to keep a recording, but it is recommended until the evaluator is experienced with the scoring procedures.

What Are the CSBS DP Materials?

The CSBS DP test kit includes:

- *CSBS DP Manual, First Normed Edition*
- Record forms for the CSBS DP Infant-Toddler Checklist, CSBS DP Caregiver Questionnaire, and CSBS DP Behavior Sample

- Carrying bag and materials for the Behavior Sample (these materials are a subset of those contained in the CSBS kit)
- Two tutorial videotapes for the Behavior Sample that contain six typically developing children; these tutorials demonstrate the sampling procedures and provide an opportunity for evaluators to practice scoring procedures.

IMPORTANT FEATURES OF THE CSBS DP

Important features of the CSBS DP include:

1. Provision of a screening checklist (i.e., CSBS DP Infant-Toddler Checklist) to determine whether referral for a developmental evaluation is needed
2. Measurement of early prelinguistic behaviors in children that have been found to be predictors of later language development in the most current research
3. Provision of specific guidelines for collecting a spontaneous sample of communication and play behaviors using naturalistic procedures so that evaluators need not rely on elicited, evaluator-directed responses typically used on formal tests
4. Measures of seven cluster areas based on information derived from both parent report and a face-to-face evaluation
5. Display of evaluation results in social, speech, and symbolic composites such that a child's social-communicative behavior can be documented in reference to his or her developmental level of expressive speech/language and symbolic representation
6. Presentation of guidelines for early identification of communication disorders and for decision making regarding areas that need assessment for program planning

For Evaluators Familiar with the CSBS, Normed Edition

For those familiar with the CSBS, Normed Edition (Wetherby & Prizant, 1993), the CSBS DP was adapted from it and uses many similar evaluation and scoring procedures. For evaluators unfamiliar with the CSBS, Normed Edition, a brief overview is given on page 5. Decisions on changes in sampling and scoring procedures for the CSBS DP were based on an effort to balance brevity and sensitivity for the purpose of early identification. Following are major features of the CSBS DP that differ from the CSBS, Normed Edition:

1. The CSBS DP Caregiver Questionnaire uses multiple-choice or recognition format, rather than the open-ended questions soliciting descriptions and examples used in the CSBS. In addition to the Caregiver Questionnaire, the CSBS DP includes a screening checklist (Infant-Toddler Checklist) to determine whether a child should be referred for an evaluation.
2. The CSBS DP Behavior Sample is much shorter than the sample used in the CSBS and consists of four communicative temptations: one book, a feeding play set, language comprehension probes, and stacking blocks. The sample is designed

Overview of CSBS, Normed Edition

The CSBS, Normed Edition (Wetherby & Prizant, 1993), is a standardized assessment tool designed to examine communicative, social-affective, and symbolic abilities of children whose functional communication age is between 8 months and 2 years. The CSBS was designed to assess infants, toddlers, and preschool children and may be used with children whose chronological age ranges from about 9 months to 5–6 years. The purpose of the CSBS is, first, for early identification of children who have or are at risk for developing a communication impairment and, second, for establishing a profile of communication, social-affective, and symbolic functioning to monitor changes in a child's behavior over time and to inform intervention planning. The CSBS measures the following parameters, summarized in seven cluster scores:

- Communicative Functions
- Gestural Communicative Means
- Vocal Communicative Means
- Verbal Communicative Means
- Reciprocity
- Social-Affective Signaling
- Symbolic Behavior

The CSBS uses two sources of information:

1. CSBS Caregiver Questionnaire, which consists of open-ended questions for parents to describe how their child displays affect; communicates with gestures, sounds, and words; and uses objects (this form can be mailed to caregivers in advance)
2. CSBS Behavior Sample, which consists of a standard, but flexible, format for sampling behavior from developmentally young children

The CSBS Behavior Sample entails the following steps, which are designed to encourage spontaneous behavior. The steps range in degree of structure provided by the adults.

- Communicative temptations, which are situations designed to entice a child to communicate
- Book sharing
- Symbolic play, using materials that encourage pretending with objects
- Language comprehension probes
- Constructive play, using materials that encourage building with objects
- Caregiver perception rating, for the caregiver to rate how typical the child's behavior was during the sample

The CSBS provides quantitative and qualitative information about a child's communicative, social-affective, and symbolic abilities. It is necessary to videotape the behavior sample to conduct the in-depth scoring procedures. The in-depth scoring method of the CSBS is both a norm-referenced and criterion-referenced measure that requires a very fine-grained analysis of communicative acts and symbolic behaviors. The results of the CSBS Behavior Sample are converted to scores on 22 five-point scales. Some scales are developmentally organized and measure performance that is expected and increases between 8 and 24 months. Other scales provide qualitative information concerning the child's behavior during the assessment.

so that it can be scored during the evaluation and includes an additional communicative temptation and book interspersed during the sample as scoring opportunities. The language comprehension probes include object names, person names, and body parts and evaluate only single-word comprehension.

3. The CSBS DP Behavior Sample scoring procedures are based on the same definitions used in the CSBS but use judgments about the presence or absence of behaviors during each sampling opportunity, rather than ratings of each communicative act.
4. The CSBS DP Behavior Sample measures 20 scales of social communication, expressive speech/language, and symbolic behavior, 19 of which were derived from the CSBS. One new scale was added—gaze/point following—and the following scales from the CSBS were not included: sociability of communicative functions, coordination of gestures and vocalizations, vocal acts without gestures, multisyllables, respondent acts, repair strategies, and negative affect.

ORGANIZATION OF THE CSBS DP MANUAL

This manual presents background on the development of the CSBS DP and specific instructions for administering, scoring, and interpreting the CSBS DP. Chapter 2 provides a description of the theoretical and empirical literature that was the basis for the development of the CSBS DP. Specific instructions for administering and scoring the CSBS DP Infant-Toddler Checklist, the CSBS DP Caregiver Questionnaire, and the CSBS DP Behavior Sample are presented in Chapters 3, 4, and 5, respectively. Chapter 6 is a self-tutorial on the sampling and scoring procedures for the Behavior Sample. This self-tutorial accompanies the CSBS DP tutorial videotapes. Chapter 7 provides the technical background and information about the standardization and norming of the CSBS DP. Finally, Chapter 8 provides guidelines for interpreting a child's CSBS DP for screening and evaluation.

DEVELOPMENT 2

The development of the CSBS DP was stimulated by the need to bridge the gap between current developmental literature and available standardized evaluation tools for young children. The national priority of early identification and intervention is reflected in the Education of the Handicapped Act Amendments of 1986 (PL 99-457) and the Individuals with Disabilities Education Act (IDEA) Amendments of 1991 (PL 102-119) and 1997 (PL 105-117). This legislation establishes a provision of funds to states choosing to develop and implement early identification and intervention services for infants and toddlers at high risk for or with a developmental delay from birth up to their third birthday, including children with delays in speech and language development. However, the early identification of children with communication or language disorders has posed a dilemma. The first symptom attended to by parents and professionals may be a delay in or failure to acquire language when other significant disabilities are not present. Because the normal range of first word acquisition is between 12 and 20 months of age, a child may not be referred for a language delay until at best 20–24 months but more typically after 30 months, especially in the absence of significant medical risks, cognitive impairments, or physical disabilities.

DEFINITION OF ASSESSMENT AND EVALUATION

The popular definition of *assessment* is the measurement of a child's knowledge, abilities, and achievement (Meisels, 1996). No clear boundary exists between assessment and intervention, but rather, assessment should be viewed as part of the intervention process. The purpose of assessment for young children is twofold: first, to identify or rule out the existence of a language or communication problem, and second, to understand the nature of the language problem in order to guide intervention decisions. The regulations stipulated in IDEA, however, distinguish between the terms *evaluation* and *assessment.*

Evaluation refers to the process used to determine a child's initial and continuing eligibility for services and includes screening, developmental evaluation, and diagnostic evaluation. Screening is the process of referral and identification of children who are at risk or high risk for developmental delays or disabilities or need an evaluation. Developmental evaluation is the process of confirming the presence or absence of a delay or disability and determining eligibility for services. Diagnostic evaluation is a more in-depth process of examining the nature of or classification of developmental delay or disability. IDEA requires that a multidisciplinary evaluation be used to determine initial eligibility of infants and toddlers for early intervention services.

Assessment refers to the ongoing procedures used to document the child's unique strengths and needs as well as the family's concerns, priorities, and resources regarding the child's development in order to plan intervention services (Crais, 1995). An assessment should provide information about a child's relative knowledge of specific skills across domains as well as guidelines for planning intervention. The tools and strategies used for evaluation will likely differ substantially from those used for assessment. Traditionally, an evaluation is conducted in a brief period of time using standardized, norm-referenced instruments. Assessment procedures usually entail multiple strategies and sources of information using criterion-referenced or curricular-based instruments and are ongoing.

WHY IS EARLY IDENTIFICATION IMPORTANT?

There is mounting evidence that intervention beginning during infancy or preschool has a greater impact on outcomes for children and families than providing services at school age (Barnett & Escobar, 1990). It is estimated that every dollar spent on early intervention can save $7.16 in later special education, crime, welfare, and other costs (Florida Starting Points, 1997). Despite federal mandates for early intervention, limitations in the identification process diminish children's access to services, and educators are not reaching most of the children and families who need help as early as they should (Meisels & Wasik, 1990). According to the 22nd Annual Report to Congress, 11% of school-age children received special education services (U.S. Department of Education, 2000). In contrast, only 4.9% of preschool children received special education, and only 1.6% of infants and toddlers received early intervention services. These statistics indicate a significant need to improve early identification of children who are likely to require special education at school age.

Brain Research

Recent advances in brain research show how the environment sculpts the young child's brain, as neurons form connections and mature in response to stimulation. The environment has the greatest potential to influence a child's developing brain during the first few years of life. Early experiences affect brain structure because the brain operates on a "use it or lose it" principle (Carnegie Task Force on Meeting the Needs of Young Children, 1994; Ounce of Prevention Fund, 1996). If a child does not have adequate emotional, physical, cognitive, and language stimulation, neurons can be lost permanently.

School Readiness

Language development is one of the most critical school readiness skills. Children's capacity to talk and the size of their vocabulary when they enter kindergarten is predictive of success in school. Children with language problems in preschool are likely to face poor educational achievement at school age and are at increased risk to develop emotional and behavioral disorders (Baker & Cantwell, 1987; Prizant et al., 1990). Follow-up studies of preschoolers with speech and language problems consistently demonstrate persisting communication impairments in a substantial proportion of children and a high incidence of learning disabilities (Howlin & Rutter, 1987). Early intervention may prevent or decrease the severity of language delays in preschoolers, enhance school readiness, and increase later academic success in school.

Cumulative Effects of Poverty and Environmental Risk

Research on young children raised in poverty demonstrates the dramatic detrimental impact that impoverished environments can have on a child's capacity to learn to talk. Strong correlations exist among the amount of time that parents talk to their children, socioeconomic status, children's vocabulary, and children's IQ scores (Hart & Risley, 1992; Walker, Greenwood, Hart, & Carta, 1994). As documented by Hart and Risley (1992), children's capacity for learning language is solidified by age 3, and the cumulative effects of the environment are evident. By school age, children in poverty are more likely to have developmental disabilities and behavior problems and to require special education services than other children (Brooks-Gunn & Duncan, 1997; U.S. Department of Education, 2000). Educational programs beginning at 3–4 years of age cannot hope to overcome such vast differences in cumulative experience. Educators are challenged to find ways to intervene very early in children's lives to effectively enhance child development and affect school readiness.

LIMITATIONS OF FORMAL TOOLS

Although there has been a proliferation of research in infant communication and socioemotional development (Prizant & Wetherby, 1990), most formal tools used for evaluation and assessment of a child's communication and language have major limitations in their capacity to evaluate a child's spontaneous communication during natural interactions. Practitioners are faced with the challenge of identifying appropriate assessment instruments for young children to meet the goals of evaluation for early identification and assessment for intervention planning. Crais (1995) and Wetherby and Prizant (1992) identified several major limitations of the most frequently used formal communication assessment instruments for young children based on current theories of language development.

First, most formal instruments emphasize language milestones and forms of communication (e.g., number of different gestures, sounds, words, word combinations), rather than the social-communicative and symbolic foundations of language. Second, most instruments involving direct child assessment are primarily clinician directed, placing the child in a respondent role and limiting observations of spontaneous, child-initiated communication. Third, most instruments do not allow for the family to collaborate in decision making about the assessment process or to participate to the extent desired by the family; therefore, they are not family-centered. There is a critical need to move toward child-centered and family-centered assessment with infants, toddlers, and developmentally young children to ensure that evaluation and assessment practices yield meaningful measures.

In order to measure a child's communicative competence in natural interactions, language sampling has become widely used to supplement formal language tools for children who engage in conversation. Similarly, communication sampling can be used to supplement formal instruments for children functioning at preverbal or early verbal stages (Wetherby, Cain, Yonclas, & Walker, 1988; Wetherby & Prizant, 1989). The CSBS (precurser to the CSBS DP) was originally conceived as an informal procedure for sampling communication with preverbal children and was standardized and normed in response to the need for more naturalistic formal assessment measures. The implementation of IDEA makes it even more critical for clinicians to develop communication-sampling procedures to evaluate very young children.

HOW CAN WE FIND CHILDREN EARLIER?

A child's level of communication development may be the best indicator of a developmental delay. Delays or disorders in communication development are the most prevalent symptom in children with disabilities (Wetherby & Prizant, 1996). When serious health or physical impairments are not present, a delay in language development may be the first evident symptom that a child is not developing typically. A language delay may be the primary problem or reflect delays in other domains (i.e., socioemotional, cognitive, motor, sensory).

There is a growing body of research indicating that prelinguistic abilities predict later language abilities. By their first birthday, children usually do not produce true words but can share attention and emotion and communicate intentionally using a variety of gestures and speech-like sounds that have shared meanings with caregivers (Bates, 1976; Bates, O'Connell, & Shore, 1987; Stern, 1985). The readability of children's signals, coupled with contingent social responsiveness, facilitates successful acquisition of communication (Dunst, Lowe, & Bartholomew, 1990; Tronick, 1989). Typically, by their second birthday children use and understand hundreds of words, construct sentences, and engage in simple conversations. Linguistic communication begins when vocabulary growth accelerates, typically at about 19 months (Bates et al., 1987; Bloom, 1993). The dramatic changes in language abilities that occur from 1 to 2 years are reflected in the transition from prelinguistic to linguistic communication.

Although most children develop their first words between 12 and 15 months, it is common practice to wait until a child is at best 18–24 months, but usually at least 30 months of age and still not talking, to refer the child for an evaluation. The challenge for service providers determining whether to make a referral for a developmental evaluation is twofold. First, many children who are late in talking catch up on their own and need to be distinguished from children who will have persistent language problems. Second, children with delayed language skills need to be identified even earlier before language develops.

There is wide variation in the age and rate of acquisition of linguistic communication; however, this variation is strongly associated with prelinguistic development. A strong association has been found between children's prelinguistic gestures and sounds, communicative functions, comprehension of words, and use of objects in play at 1 year and language skills at 2 and 3 years (Paul, 1991; Paul & Jennings, 1992; Paul, Looney, & Dahm, 1991; Rescorla & Goosens, 1992; Thal & Tobias, 1992; Thal, Tobias, & Morrison, 1991; Wetherby et al., 1988). Many children are late in learning to talk, and many of these children do not need early intervention services. About 15% of 24-month-olds are late talkers with no other obvious delays (i.e., having fewer than 50 words or no word combinations; Rescorla, 1989, 1991). About half of these children show persisting problems in language development at age 3; the other half catch up with their peers spontaneously without intervention (Paul, 1991; Rescorla & Schwartz, 1990; Thal et al., 1991).

Research on preschoolers with language delays has important implications for distinguishing between children who will catch up spontaneously from those whose language problems are likely to persist. (For a review of this research, see McCathren, Warren, & Yoder, 1996; Olswang, Rodriguez, & Timler, 1998; Wetherby & Prizant, 1992.) These studies have identified a collection of language predictors that are prelinguistic indicators of later language development and promise earlier and more accurate identification. The following seven language predictors have been identified:

1. Emotion and eye gaze
2. Rate and function of communication
3. Use of gestures
4. Use of sounds
5. Use of words
6. Understanding of words
7. Use of objects

These studies have demonstrated that children delayed only in the use of words are very likely to catch up on their own while children who are delayed also in several or many of the other predictors are likely to have persisting problems. Instead of waiting for children to start using words, evaluating these language predictors is a promising solution to improve early identification.

The literature reviewed previously suggests that a child's profile of communicative and symbolic abilities, even prior to the emergence of words, may be a sensitive indicator of the likelihood of subsequent difficulties in communication and language development. The findings for young children who show persisting language impairments indicate that measures of vocabulary alone are insufficient for early identification. Multiple measures across communicative and symbolic domains are necessary for earlier identification and differentiation of children who will outgrow their delay, from those children who have specific versus more pervasive social or cognitive impairments. That is, a child who shows expressive language delays at 2 years and also shows delays in one or more of the other language predictors would be at a much higher risk than a child who demonstrates expressive language delays only.

These findings suggest greater urgency in initiating intervention that addresses delays, not only in expressive language, but also in other communicative and symbolic parameters. Because it is not yet possible to consider delays in expressive language for children younger than 18 months, it is even more critical to measure other parameters of communication and symbolic development in children younger than 18 months. Furthermore, patterns of strengths and weaknesses in the language predictors should provide critical information contributing to the early identification of a developmental disability. This empirical and theoretical framework forms the basis of the CSBS DP.

DEVELOPMENT OF THE CSBS DP

The CSBS DP was designed to measure the seven language predictors using multiple sources of information to screen and evaluate very young children. The CSBS DP Infant-Toddler Checklist and CSBS DP Caregiver Questionnaire were adapted from the CSBS Caregiver Questionnaire (Wetherby & Prizant, 1993) and research on the MacArthur Communicative Development Inventories (CDI; Fenson et al., 1993, 1994). The CSBS DP Infant-Toddler Checklist and CSBS DP Caregiver Questionnaire were designed for caregivers to be able to report accurately and efficiently. Several studies indicate that the use of parent report is a reliable and valid measure of communication development as well as a sensitive indicator of language delays in young children (Bates, Bretherton, & Snyder, 1988; Dale, Bates, Reznick, & Morisset, 1989; Fenson et al., 1994; Rescorla, 1989; 1991).

Research on parent report has demonstrated that parents can be very accurate in reporting about current and emerging behaviors, as opposed to giving retrospective accounts of past milestones. Furthermore, the accuracy is greater when a recognition format or checklist is used instead of free-form reports or diary methods (Fenson et al., 1993). For these reasons, we have chosen to use a recognition format for the CSBS DP Caregiver Questionnaire. Most of the items included are based on normative data from the CSBS, Normed Edition (Wetherby & Prizant, 1993), and are included to gather information about the same parameters measured with the CSBS DP Behavior Sample. The recognition list for words used and words understood were derived from the research findings of Fenson et al. (1994) on the first 36 words reported with the highest frequency by parents with the MacArthur CDI, which is a more extensive checklist of vocabulary and communicative development.

The CSBS DP Behavior Sample was derived from the CSBS Behavior Sample (Wetherby & Prizant, 1993) and was modified by reducing the length of the sample but maintaining the naturalistic quality of the interaction. The scoring procedures were modified by reducing the number of scales from 22 to 20 and simplifying the method for scoring in order to enable the evaluator to rate the behavior during the sample or very quickly from videotape.

Our decisions regarding modifying the sampling and scoring procedures were based on research on children with and without communication impairments (Wetherby & Prizant, 1993; Wetherby, Prizant, & Hutchinson, 1998). Nineteen of the twenty scales were derived from the CSBS. One new scale was added, gaze/point following, based on the findings of Mundy, Kasari, Sigman, and Ruskin (1995). These decisions were made in an effort to include scales that were most critical for early identification. Limiting the sampling and scoring procedures reduced the amount of administration and scoring time to a clinically feasible evaluation tool. The parameters measured on the CSBS DP Behavior Sample are defined in Table 2.1

Table 2.1. Twenty scales measured with the CSBS DP Behavior Sample

Emotion and Eye Gaze

1. *Gaze shifts*—alternating eye gaze between a person and an object and back (i.e., person–object–person or object–person–object)
2. *Shared positive affect*—clear facial expression of pleasure or excitement directed toward other with eye gaze
3. *Gaze/point following*—responding to another's gaze/point by turning head or following with eye gaze

Communication

4. *Rate of communicating*—frequency of communicative acts displayed per sampling opportunity
5. *Behavior regulation*—use of communication to regulate behavior of another to obtain or restrict an environmental goal
6. *Social interaction*—use of communication to attract attention to self
7. *Joint attention*—use of communication to direct another's attention to an object or event

Gestures

8. *Conventional gestures*—repertoire of gestural communication with shared or conventional meaning, including giving, showing, pushing/pulling away, reaching, pointing, waving, nodding head, and shaking head
9. *Distal gestures*—gestural communicative acts in which the child's hand does not touch a person or object (e.g., open-hand reaching, pointing at a distance, waving)

Sounds

10. *Syllables with consonants*—vocal communicative acts that are transcribable vowel plus consonant combinations
11. *Inventory of consonants*—the variety of different consonants produced in communicative acts

Words

12. *Words*—use of words (i.e., spoken or signed) in communicative acts; a word or word approximation must be used to refer to a specific object, action, or attribute and only that word class
13. *Inventory of words*—sample of different words used (i.e., spoken or signed) in communicative acts
14. *Word combinations*—use of multiword combinations in communicative acts
15. *Inventory of word combinations*—sample of different word combinations used in communicative acts

Understanding

16. *Language comprehension*—comprehension of object names, person names, and body parts

Object Use

17. *Inventory of action schemes*—the variety of different action schemes used with objects in symbolic play
18. *Action schemes toward other*—the use of action schemes with objects toward other agents in pretend play
19. *Action schemes in sequence*—the use of action schemes with objects in sequence of different action schemes in pretend play
20. *Constructive play*—the use of objects in combination to construct a product; that is, to stack a tower of blocks

CSBS DP INFANT-TODDLER CHECKLIST

3

The first step in the CSBS DP two-step process is screening with the CSBS DP Infant-Toddler Checklist, as diagramed in Figure 3.1.

ADMINISTRATION PROCEDURES

The CSBS DP Infant-Toddler Checklist is a screening tool designed to determine whether a referral for a developmental evaluation is needed. As with the other components of the CSBS DP, the checklist measures the following seven language predictors:

- Emotion and eye gaze
- Communication
- Gestures
- Sounds
- Words
- Understanding
- Object use

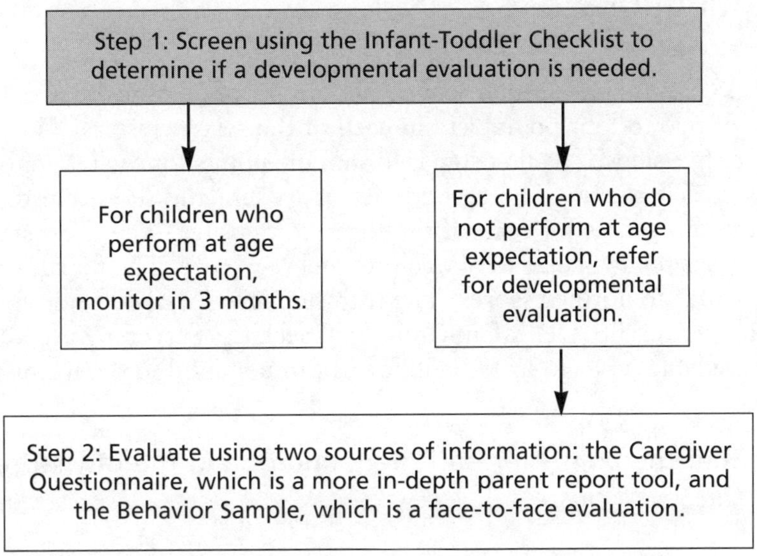

Figure 3.1. First step in the CSBS DP two-step process.

The CSBS DP Infant-Toddler Checklist is the first step in routine developmental screening for children ages 6–24 months to decide if a developmental evaluation is needed. The CSBS DP Infant-Toddler Checklist consists of 24 items; families select from three to five choices for each item. It is designed to accompany the CSBS DP Infant-Toddler Checklist: Family Information Form. The CSBS DP Infant-Toddler Checklist: Family Information Form is used to collect 1) family contact information for follow-up, 2) information on birth and health history, and 3) a description of any concerns about the child's development.

The CSBS DP Infant-Toddler Checklist and CSBS DP Infant-Toddler Checklist: Family Information Form can be given to families in pediatricians' offices during well-child checkups or routine visits, in child care centers, or in other facilities serving infants and toddlers and their families. They should be given to any family of a child between the ages of 6 and 24 months, regardless of whether that family has a concern about their child's development. The Checklist is to be completed by a caregiver, who may be either a parent or another person who nurtures the child on a daily basis. It takes about 5–10 minutes to complete. For caregivers who cannot answer the questions by reading them or writing the responses, the questions may be presented in an interview format with adequate explanations to clarify what is being asked. It is recommended that the Checklist be used to monitor development every 3 months between 6 and 24 months of age.

The Checklist can be used independently or along with the other components of the CSBS DP. The Checklist is copyrighted (Brookes, 2002) but remains free for use and can be downloaded from the Internet and freely photocopied or duplicated by other methods. Files that include the Infant-Toddler Checklist and the Infant-Toddler Checklist: Family Information Form are available from Paul H. Brookes Publishing Co. at http://www.brookespublishing.com/csbsdp. They also are available at the FIRST WORDS Project web site, http://firstwords.fsu.edu. The Checklist is to be completed by families or other caregivers but should be scored by health care or child care service providers.

SCORING INSTRUCTIONS

The CSBS DP Infant-Toddler Checklist consists of 24 items that range from a total possible of two to four points within each of the seven clusters. The scoring process consists of five steps. The first step is to sum the points for each item to obtain the raw scores for each cluster. The second step is to sum the seven cluster raw scores to obtain the raw scores for each of the three composites. The third step is to add the three composite raw scores to obtain the total raw score. The fourth step is to convert the raw scores to normed scores. The fifth step is to interpret and report the normed scores on the CSBS DP Infant-Toddler Checklist: Screening Report. An example form is available on page 130. Blank forms can be found in the forms packet.

Step 1: Sum the points for each item and obtain the raw scores for each of the seven clusters.

Give credit of 0 points for items checked *Not Yet*, 1 point for items checked *Sometimes*, or 2 points for items checked *Often*. For items that describe a series of numbers or ranges, give credit of 0 points for items checked *None* and 1–4 points for items containing numbered choices. That is, for Items 16 and 22, give credit of 0 points for *None*, 1 point for *1–2*, 2 points for *3–4*, 3 points for *5–8*, and 4 points for *Over 8*. For Items 17 and 20, give credit of 0 points for *None*, 1 point for *1–3*, 2 points for *4–10*, 3 points for *11–30*, and 4 points for *Over 30*. For Item 23, give credit of 0 points for *None*, 1 point for *2 blocks*, 2 points for *3–4 blocks*, 3 points for *5 or more blocks*. The point values and total possible points for each item are listed in Table 3.1.

The number of points earned in each cluster should be totaled to yield raw scores. The seven cluster raw scores can be tallied on the CSBS DP Infant-Toddler Checklist to the right of the label for each cluster and then transferred to the left side of the column labeled *Raw Score* on the CSBS DP Infant-Toddler Checklist: Screening Report. Refer to page 130. The total possible points for the seven cluster raw scores are listed in Table 3.2.

Step 2: Sum the seven cluster raw scores to obtain the raw scores for each of the three composites.

The seven clusters are organized into three composites—Social, Speech, and Symbolic.

The second step is to sum the seven cluster raw scores to obtain the three composite raw scores. On the CSBS DP Infant-Toddler Checklist: Screening Report, the seven cluster raw scores should be summed to yield the raw scores for the three composites. That is, the raw score for the Social composite is the sum of the Emotion and Eye Gaze, Communication, and Gestures Clusters. The raw score for the Speech Composite is the sum of the Sounds and Words Clusters. The raw score for the Symbolic Composite is the sum of the Understanding and Object Use Clusters. The composite raw scores should be tallied on the right side of the column labeled *Raw Score* on the Infant-Toddler Checklist: Screening Report. The total possible points for the three composite raw scores are listed in Table 3.2.

Table 3.1. Point values and total possible points of each item on the Infant-Toddler Checklist

Cluster	Number of items	Possible points	Total possible
Emotion and Eye Gaze			
Items 1-4	4	2	8
Communication			
Items 5-8	4	2	8
Gestures			
Items 9-13	5	2	10
Sounds			
Items 14-15	2	2	4
Item 16	1	4	4
Words			
Item 17	1	4	4
Item 18	1	2	2
Understanding			
Item 19	1	2	2
Item 20	1	4	4
Object Use			
Item 21	1	2	2
Item 22	1	4	4
Item 23	1	3	3
Item 24	1	2	2

Table 3.2. Total possible points for each cluster, composite, and total on the Infant-Toddler Checklist

Composite	Possible Points
Social Composite	
Emotion and Eye Gaze	8
Communication	8
Gestures	10
Total	**26**
Speech Composite	
Sounds	8
Words	6
Total	**14**
Symbolic Composite	
Understanding	6
Object Use	11
Total	**17**
Social Composite	26
Speech Composite	14
Symbolic Composite	17
Total	**57**

Step 3: Sum the three composite raw scores to obtain the total raw score.

The third step is to sum the three composite raw scores to obtain the total raw score. On the CSBS DP Infant-Toddler Checklist: Screening Report, the three composite raw scores should be summed to yield the total raw score. The total raw score should be tallied on the right side of the column labeled *Raw Score* on the Infant-Toddler Checklist: Screening Report, just below the composite raw scores. The total possible points for the total raw score are listed in Table 3.2.

Step 4: Convert the composite and total raw scores to normed scores.

The fourth step is to convert the composite and total raw scores to normed scores. Normed scores are provided in the norms tables for the CSBS DP Infant-Toddler Checklist in Appendix A and are based on chronological age to reflect the performance of children in the standardization sample by 1-month intervals from 6 to 24 months.

Use the following steps to compute the child's chronological age:

1. Enter the child's name, date filled out, and date of birth on the CSBS DP Infant-Toddler Checklist: Screening Report. If the child is more than 4 weeks premature, make sure to enter the child's corrected date of birth and indicate this by writing *corrected* in parentheses after the date of birth and chronological age.
2. If the child is more than 4 weeks premature, compute the child's chronological age on the CSBS DP Infant-Toddler Checklist: Screening Report by subtracting the child's date of birth or corrected date of birth (month, day, and year) from the date of completion (month, day, and year).
3. Subtract days first, then months, then years. Table 3.3 shows a simple subtraction in which no borrowing is required.
4. If the day of the month on which the child was born is larger than the day of the month of testing, borrow 30 days; that is, add 30 days to the day of testing and

Table 3.3. Calculating chronological age without needing to borrow

	Month	Day	Year
Date of completion	10	25	2000
Date of birth	6	4	1999
Chronological age	**4**	**21**	**1**
CSBS DP age	**16**		

Table 3.4. Calculating chronological age with borrowing

	Month	Day	Year
Date of completion	~~11~~ 10	~~5~~ 35	2000
Date of birth	1	28	2000
Chronological age	**9**	**7**	**0**
CSBS DP age	**9**		

subtract 1 month from the month of testing. If necessary, also borrow 1 month of testing by adding 12 months to the actual month of testing and subtracting 1 year from the testing year. Table 3.4 shows a subtraction in which borrowing is required to calculate chronological age for a child whose date of completion was November 5, 2000.

5. The child's chronological age should be reported in months, and the month should not be rounded up. For example, a child is 12 months old from 12 months and 0 days until that child turns 13 months and 0 days. To calculate age in months, first multiply the number of years by 12, and then add the number of extra months. The chronological age for the child in Table 3.3 is 16 months (i.e., multiply 1 for the number of years by 12 and add 4 extra months to get 16) and would not be rounded to 17 months, even though the child is more than $16\frac{1}{2}$ months old. The chronological age for the child in Table 3.4 is 9 months.

Standard scores and percentile ranks are the normed scores provided in the norms tables for the composites and total of the CSBS DP Infant-Toddler Checklist in Appendix A. The standard scores for the three composites are based on a mean of 10 and a standard deviation of 3. The standard scores for the total are based on a mean of 100 and a standard deviation of 15. Because standard scores reflect equal units of measurement, they may be added, subtracted, or averaged. A percentile rank reflects the percentage of children in the sample scoring at or below a given raw score. Percentile ranks, unlike standard scores, should not be added, subtracted, or averaged. Standard scores, rather than percentile ranks, should be used to reflect average performance, whether it is the average of several scores for an individual child or the average of scores obtained from a group of children. The relationship between the standard scores for the composites and total and percentile ranks is shown in Table 3.5.

Table 3.5. Standard deviations (SD), standard scores (SS), and percentile ranks (%ile) for the composites and total scores

SD	Composite SS	Total SS	%ile
	17	135	99
+2 SD	16	130	98
	15	125	95
	14	120	91
+1 SD	13	115	84
	12	110	75
	11	105	63
Mean	10	100	50
	9	95	37
	8	90	25
–1 SD	7	85	16
	6	80	9
	5	75	5
–2 SD	4	70	2
	3	65	1

Once the child's chronological age is known, use the following steps to look up the standard scores and percentile ranks for the composite and total raw scores.

1. Use the norms tables for the CSBS DP Infant-Toddler Checklist in Appendix A. On the table for the Social Composite, find the column with the child's chronological age in months, read down the column until you find the child's Social Composite raw score and look to the left to find the corresponding standard score (SS) and percentile (%ile) rank. Enter these scores in the appropriate columns on the CSBS DP Infant-Toddler Checklist: Screening Report.
2. Repeat this for the Speech Composite, the Symbolic Composite, and the total raw scores.

Step 5: Interpret and report the normed scores on the CSBS DP Infant-Toddler Checklist: Screening Report.

The fifth and last step is to interpret and report the normed scores on the CSBS DP Infant-Toddler Checklist: Screening Report. Once the child's standard scores and percentile ranks are entered, use the following steps to determine if the normed scores are of concern and to decide what to recommend.

1. Determine if the normed scores are of concern and enter *Yes* in the column labeled *Concern*. Leave blank if child is at or above criterion level. Four scores may fall in a range of concern or no concern—the three composite scores and the total score. We have set the criterion level for concern for the composite and total scores based on performance of at least 1.25 standard deviations below the mean as follows:
   - Standard scores at or below 6 for the composite scores
   - Standard scores at or below 81 for the total score
   - Percentile ranks at or below the 10th for the composites and total scores
2. Make a recommendation on the bottom of the CSBS DP Infant-Toddler Checklist: Screening Report by checking one of the three boxes. Based on our validation studies summarized in Chapter 7, we have determined that the following recommendation should be made, depending on the child's pattern of scores:
   - A child should be referred for an evaluation if the Social Composite, Symbolic Composite, *or* the total score are in the concern range.
   - A child should be monitored carefully if the Speech Composite is in the concern range and should be referred for an evaluation if in the concern range on a second Checklist completed 3 months later.

It is recommended that the Checklist be used to monitor development every 3 months between 6 and 24 months of age. Because it is based on parent report, it is possible for the caregiver to overestimate or underestimate the child's abilities. Therefore, this tool should be used along with a brief observation of the child by a health care or child care service provider. Children who have scores in the concern range on any composite or the total score may have specific language impairments, hearing impairments, more general developmental delays, or autism spectrum disorder. With further development, they may only have speech impairments or they may catch up to children their age. The Checklist should only be used to decide that a developmental evaluation is needed.

Caution should be taken not to alarm parents. We find that many parents already have concerns about their child, especially as their child is approaching age 18 months and is behind in language development. The early intervention literature emphasizes the notion of multiple risk factors; therefore, a child's scores on this Checklist need to be considered in relation to other known biological or environmental risk factors. Clinical judgment should be used in making decisions about the need for further evaluation with these cutoffs as guidelines. Remember that the Checklist is not meant for a diagnostic evaluation and should not be used for a differential diagnosis.

COMPUTER SCORING OF THE CHECKLIST

A computer software program for use with the Checklist is available from Paul H. Brookes Publishing Co. (800-638-3775; www.brookespublishing.com). Users input the child's name, date of birth, and date the Checklist was filled out and select the responses to the 24 questions of the CSBS DP Infant-Toddler Checklist from a menu. The program calculates the raw scores, standard scores, and percentile ranks for the cluster scores, composite scores, and the total score. The program also can print a CSBS DP Infant-Toddler Checklist: Screening Report that includes a table with the raw scores, standard scores, and percentile ranks along with a matching parent letter summarizing the screening recommendation.

CSBS DP CAREGIVER QUESTIONNAIRE

4

The second step in the CSBS DP two-step process is evaluating with the CSBS DP Caregiver Questionnaire and CSBS DP Behavior Sample, as diagramed in Figure 4.1. This chapter explains how to administer the CSBS DP Caregiver Questionnaire and provides instructions for scoring the questionnaire and for completing the CSBS DP Caregiver Questionnaire: Scoring Worksheet and the CSBS DP Caregiver Questionnaire: Scoring Summary. All of these forms are available in the forms packet.

ADMINISTRATION PROCEDURES

The CSBS DP Caregiver Questionnaire is an evaluation tool based on parent report. It was designed as a more in-depth follow-up to the CSBS DP Infant-Toddler Checklist and a companion to the CSBS DP Behavior Sample to determine whether a child has a developmental delay or disability in the areas measured. As with the other components of the CSBS DP, the Caregiver Questionnaire measures the following seven language predictors:

- Emotion and eye gaze
- Communication
- Gestures
- Sounds
- Words
- Understanding
- Object use

The CSBS DP Caregiver Questionnaire can be mailed ahead or given to the caregiver in the waiting room when the child is brought in for the CSBS DP Behavior Sample. The caregiver should be either a parent or someone who nurtures the child on a daily basis. If the child has more than one caregiver, both caregivers may want to fill it out together. The questionnaire is designed to be self-explanatory for caregivers who can read. It should take about 15–20 minutes to complete. For caregivers who cannot answer the questions by reading them or writing the responses, the questions may be presented in an interview format prior to, immediately after, or on a different day than the Behavior Sample. The explanations can then be given as needed to clarify what is being asked.

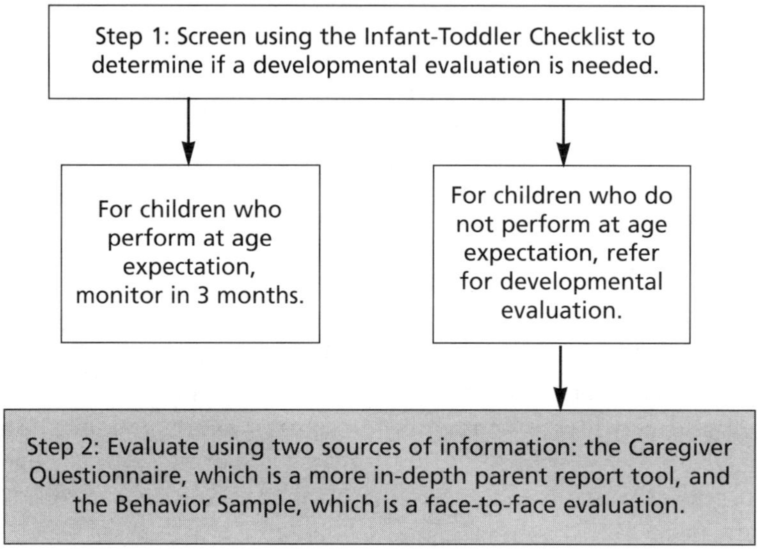

Figure 4.1. Second step in the CSBS DP two-step process.

SCORING INSTRUCTIONS

The CSBS DP Caregiver Questionnaire consists of 41 multiple-choice items within each of the seven clusters and four open-ended questions. The multiple-choice items should be scored as described next, and the responses to the open-ended questions should be examined and considered in the interpretation of results. The scoring process consists of five steps. The first step is to sum the points for each item and to compute the weighted raw scores for each cluster. The second step is to sum the seven cluster weighted raw scores to obtain the weighted raw scores for each of the three composite scores. The third step is to sum the three composite weighted raw scores to obtain the total weighted raw score. The fourth step is to convert the weighted raw scores to normed scores. The fifth step is to interpret and report the normed scores.

Step 1: Sum the points for each item, and obtain the weighted raw scores for each of the seven clusters.

Give credit of 0 points for items checked *Not Yet* or *Rarely*, 1 point for items checked *Sometimes*, or 2 points for items checked *Often* or *Usually*, with only one exception—Item 5, which is in the Emotion and Eye Gaze cluster. For Item 5, "How often does your child get upset or frustrated?" reverse the point assignment and give 0 points for *Often*, 1 point for *Sometimes*, or 2 points for *Rarely*. For items that list an inventory of skills to be checked, give credit of 0 points for items not checked and 1 point for items checked. That is, for Items 20, 23, 26, 32, 35, 37, 40, and 41, give credit of 1 point for each box checked.

The number of points earned should be totaled to yield weighted raw scores for each of the seven clusters. The items should be tallied on the CSBS DP Caregiver Questionnaire: Scoring Worksheet. Some of the items that list an inventory of skills are weighted in order to make the point value for these items and clusters comparable. In the last three clusters—Words, Understanding, and Object Use—the sum of the items needs to be weighted by dividing by 2 for Items 26, 32, 35, 37, 40, and 41. Thus, the sum of the items for the first four clusters can be tallied quickly, with special care to reverse the point value for Item 5. The sum of the items for the last three clusters should be tallied more carefully, with particular attention to dividing by 2 for the items that are weighted. Then, the weighted raw scores should be summed for each cluster and written in the shaded boxes. The point values, weighting, and total possible weighted points are listed in Table 4.1.

Step 2: Sum the seven cluster weighted raw scores to obtain the raw scores for each of the three composites.

The seven clusters are organized into three composites—Social, Speech, and Symbolic. The second step is to sum the seven weighted cluster raw scores to obtain the three weighted composite raw scores. The seven weighted cluster raw scores (tallied on the CSBS DP Caregiver Questionnaire: Scoring Worksheet) should be trans-

Table 4.1. Point values of each item, weighting, and total possible weighted points for each cluster on the Caregiver Questionnaire

Cluster	Number of items	Possible points	Weighting	Weighted points
Emotion and Eye Gaze				
Items 1–8	8	2		16
Total				**16**
Communication				
Items 9–18	10	2		20
Total				**20**
Gestures				
Item 19	1	2		2
Item 20	10	1		10
Total				**12**
Sounds				
Items 21–22	2	2		4
Item 23	10	1		10
Item 24	1	2		2
Total				**16**
Words				
Item 25	1	2		2
Item 26	36	1	Divide by 2	18
Items 27–28	2	2		4
Total				**24**
Understanding				
Items 29-31	3	2		6
Item 32	36	1	Divide by 2	18
Total				**24**
Object Use				
Items 33–34	2	2		4
Item 35	10	1	Divide by 2	5
Items 36	1	2		2
Item 37	8	1	Divide by 2	4
Items 38–39	2	2		4
Item 40	10	1	Divide by 2	5
Item 41	6	1	Divide by 2	3
Total				**27**

ferred to the left-hand column labeled *Weighted Raw Score* on the CSBS DP Caregiver Questionnaire: Scoring Summary. These seven weighted cluster raw scores should be summed to yield the weighted raw scores for the three composites. The weighted raw score for the Communication Composite is the sum of the clusters for Emotion and Eye Gaze, Communication, and Gestures. The weighted raw score for the Speech composite is the sum of the Sounds and Words Clusters. The weighted raw score for the Symbolic Composite is the sum of the clusters for Understanding and Object Use. The composite weighted raw scores should be tallied in the column labeled *Weighted Raw Score* under the cluster weighted raw scores on the CSBS DP Caregiver Questionnaire: Scoring Summary. The total possible points for the three composite raw scores are listed in Table 4.2.

Step 3: Sum the three composite weighted raw scores to obtain the total weighted raw score.

The third step is to sum the three composite weighted raw scores to obtain the total weighted raw score. On the CSBS DP Caregiver Questionnaire: Scoring Summary, the three composite weighted raw scores should be summed to yield the total weighted raw score. The total weighted raw score should be tallied in the column labeled weighted raw score on the Caregiver Questionnaire: Scoring Summary, just below the composite weighted raw scores. The total possible points for the total weighted raw score are listed in Table 4.2.

Step 4: Convert the cluster, composite, and total weighted raw scores to normed scores.

The fourth step is to convert the cluster, composite, and total weighted raw scores to normed scores. Normed scores are provided in the norms tables for the CSBS DP

Table 4.2. Total possible points for each cluster, composite and total on the Caregiver Questionnaire

Composite	Possible points
Social Composite	
Emotion and Eye Gaze	16
Communication	20
Gestures	12
Total	**48**
Speech Composite	
Sounds	16
Words	24
Total	**40**
Symbolic Composite	
Understanding	24
Object Use	27
Total	**51**
Social Composite	48
Speech Composite	40
Symbolic Composite	51
Total	**139**

Caregiver Questionnaire in Appendix B and are based on chronological age to reflect the performance of children in the standardization sample by 2-month intervals from 6 to 24 months, with the exception of 12 months, which is by a 1-month interval. Use the following steps to compute the child's chronological age:

1. Enter the child's name, date filled out, and date of birth on the CSBS DP Caregiver Questionnaire: Scoring Worksheet. If the child is more than 4 weeks premature, make sure to enter the child's corrected date of birth and indicate this by writing *corrected* in parentheses after the date of birth and chronological age.
2. If a child is more than 4 weeks premature, compute the child's chronological age on the CSBS DP Caregiver Questionnaire: Scoring Worksheet by subtracting the child's date of birth (month, day, and year) from the date of completion (month, day, and year).
3. Subtract days first, then months, then years. Table 4.3 shows a simple subtraction in which no borrowing is required.
4. If the day of the month on which the child was born is larger than the day of the month of testing, borrow 30 days; that is, add 30 days to the day of testing and subtract 1 month from the month of testing. If necessary, also borrow 1 month of testing by adding 12 months to the actual month of testing and subtracting 1 year from the testing year. Table 4.4 shows a subtraction, where borrowing is required, for a child whose date of completion was November 5, 2000.
5. The child's chronological age should be reported in months, and the month should not be rounded up. For example, a child is 12 months old from 12 months and 0 days until that child turns 13 months and 0 days. To calculate age in months, first multiply the number of years by 12, and then add the number of extra months. The chronological age for the child in Table 4.3 is 16 months (i.e., multiply 1 for the number of years by 12 and add 4 extra months to get 16) and would not be rounded to 17 months, even though the child is more than $16^1/_2$ months old. The chronological age for the child in Table 4.4 is 9 months.

Standard scores and percentile ranks are the normed scores provided in the norms tables for the clusters, composites, and total for the CSBS DP Caregiver Questionnaire in Appendix B. The standard scores for the seven clusters and three composites are based on a mean of 10 and a standard deviation of 3. The standard scores for the total are based on a mean of 100 and a standard deviation of 15. Because standard scores reflect equal units of measurement, they may be added, subtracted, or averaged. A percentile rank reflects the percentage of children in the sample scoring at or below a given raw score. Percentile ranks, unlike standard scores, should not be added, subtracted, or averaged. Standard scores, rather than

Table 4.3. Calculating chronological age without needing to borrow

	Month	Day	Year
Date of completion	10	25	2000
Date of birth	6	4	1999
Chronological age	**4**	**21**	**1**
CSBS DP age	**16**		

Table 4.4. Calculating chronological age with borrowing

	Month	Day	Year
Date of completion	~~11~~ 10	~~5~~ 35	2000
Date of birth	1	28	2000
Chronological age	**9**	**7**	**0**
CSBS DP age	**9**		

Table 4.5. Standard deviations (SD), standard scores (SS), and percentile ranks (%ile) for the clusters, composites and total scores

SD	Cluster and composite SS	Total SS	%ile
	17	135	99
+2 SD	16	130	98
	15	125	95
	14	120	91
+1 SD	13	115	84
	12	110	75
	11	105	63
Mean	10	100	50
	9	95	37
	8	90	25
–1 SD	7	85	16
	6	80	9
	5	75	5
–2 SD	4	70	2
	3	65	1

percentile ranks, should be used to reflect average performance, whether it is the average of several scores for an individual child or the average of scores obtained from a group of children. The relationship between the standard scores and percentile ranks is shown in Table 4.5.

Once the child's chronological age is known, use the following steps to look up the standard scores and percentile ranks for the clusters, composites, and total weighted raw scores.

1. Use the norms tables for the CSBS DP Caregiver Questionnaire in Appendix B. On the table for the Emotion and Eye Gaze Cluster, find the column with the child's chronological age in months, read down the column until you find the child's Emotion and Eye Gaze Cluster weighted raw score, and look to the left to find the corresponding standard score (SS) and percentile rank (%ile). Enter these scores in the appropriate columns on the CSBS DP Caregiver Questionnaire: Scoring Summary. (*Note:* If the CSBS DP Caregiver Questionnaire is being used to monitor change for children who are older than 24 months of age, use the oldest normative group, which is 23–24 months old for comparison purposes but document this when reporting results.)
2. Repeat this for the other six clusters, the three composites, and the total.

Step 5: Interpret and report the normed scores

The fifth and last step is to interpret and report the normed scores. Once the child's standard scores and percentile ranks are entered, use the following steps to determine if the normed scores are of concern and decide what to recommend.

1. Determine if the normed scores are of concern and enter *Yes* in the column labeled *Concern*. Leave blank if the area is not of concern. There are 11 scores that may fall in a range of concern or no concern—the seven clusters, the three composites, and the total. We have set the criterion level for concern for the composite and total scores based on performance of at least 1.25 standard deviations below the mean as follows:

- Standard scores at or below 6 for the clusters and composites
- Standard scores at or below 81 for the total score
- Percentile ranks at or below the 10th percentile for the composites and total scores

2. Compare the normed scores on the CSBS DP Caregiver Questionnaire with those obtained from the CSBS DP Behavior Sample (see Chapter 5 for administration guidelines).

The CSBS DP Caregiver Questionnaire can be used to monitor development every 3 months between 6 and 24 months of age. Because it is based on parent report, it is possible for the caregiver to overestimate or underestimate the child's abilities. Therefore, this tool should be used along with a face-to-face evaluation of the child. Although eligibility criteria for receiving services vary from state to state, it is recommended that children who have scores in the concern range on at least three clusters, any composite, or the total score be considered at-risk for a developmental delay or disability. If a consistent pattern is also documented on the Behavior Sample, the child should be referred for a diagnostic evaluation and/or further assessment to plan support or intervention services. If there is a discrepancy between the pattern of scores on the CSBS DP Caregiver Questionnaire and the CSBS DP Behavior Sample, reasons for this discrepancy should be considered (i.e., Is the parent over- or underestimating the child's performance or is the child performing below potential on the Behavior Sample?).

The Caregiver Questionnaire should only be used along with the Behavior Sample to decide if a child has developmental delays. Caution should be taken not to alarm parents. We find that many parents already have concerns about their children, especially if the child is about 18 months old and is behind in language development. The early intervention literature emphasizes the notion of multiple risk factors, and therefore, a child's scores on this Caregiver Questionnaire need to be considered in relation to other known biological or environmental risk factors. Clinical judgment should be used in making decisions about the need for further evaluation with these cutoffs as guidelines. Remember that the CSBS DP Caregiver Questionnaire is not meant for a diagnostic evaluation and should not be used for a differential diagnosis.

CSBS DP BEHAVIOR SAMPLE 5

The second step in the CSBS DP two-step process is evaluating with the CSBS DP Caregiver Questionnaire and CSBS DP Behavior Sample (see Figure 5.1). This chapter provides detailed descriptions of the administration procedures for gathering the CSBS DP Behavior Sample and the scoring procedures for rating behaviors. You will learn how to complete the Behavior Sample: Scoring Worksheet as well as how to fill out the CSBS DP Behavior Sample: Scoring Summary.

ADMINISTRATION PROCEDURES

The CSBS DP Behavior Sample is a face-to-face evaluation tool for professionals. It was designed as a more in-depth follow-up to the CSBS DP Infant-Toddler Checklist and a companion to the CSBS DP Caregiver Questionnaire to determine whether a child has a developmental delay or disability in the areas measured. As with the other components of the CSBS DP, the CSBS DP Behavior Sample measures the following seven language predictors:

- Emotion and eye gaze
- Communication
- Gestures
- Sounds
- Words
- Understanding
- Object use

The CSBS DP Behavior Sample can be scored while it is being collected using the CSBS Behavior Sample: Scoring Worksheet. Calculated scores are compiled on the CSBS DP Behavior Sample: Scoring Summary. The complete sampling procedures take about 30 minutes per child, including a warm-up. While it is not necessary to record the responses on videotape, some evaluators choose to record the Behavior Sample for later analysis or documentation. It is recommended that the Behavior Sample be videotaped until the evaluator is experienced with the scoring procedures.

Behaviors are sampled in different contexts, which vary in the degree of structure provided by the adult:

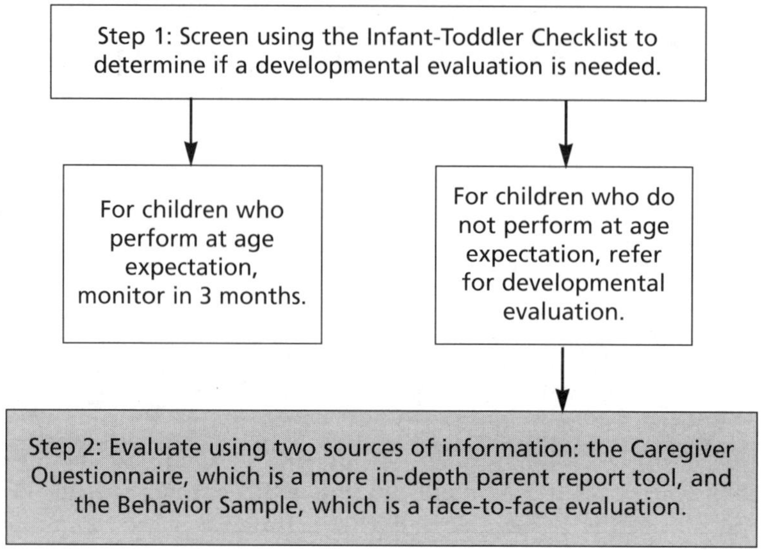

Figure 5.1. Second step in the CSBS DP two-step process.

1. Warm-up 2–10 minutes
2. Communicative temptations 5–10 minutes
3. Book sharing 2 minutes
4. Symbolic play probe 5 minutes
5. Language comprehension probe 2 minutes
6. Constructive play probe 1 minute

The times indicated are estimates and should be used as guidelines to set the pace of the interaction.

The child's caregiver should be present during the entire session. Ask the caregiver to react naturally to the child's communicative behavior but to avoid directing the child's behavior (as specified in the instructions below for each context). Throughout the sampling session, the evaluator should speak predominantly in response to the child's communicative behavior. That is, the evaluator should talk after the child has focused attention on an object or event or has initiated a verbal or nonverbal communicative act. Respond to the child's act by interpreting, acknowledging, imitating, expanding, or extending. Try not to ask questions except to request clarification or further information. It is important for the evaluator and caregiver to talk enough but not too much. If the adults do not talk enough, the child may be less likely to vocalize or use words. If the adults talk too much or direct the child with instructions and questions, the child may be less likely to initiate communication.

Behavior Sample Environment

Administer the CSBS DP Behavior Sample in a room set up for that purpose, where there is no other activity to distract the child. If possible, use a small room and make sure there are a few interesting things (e.g., pictures on the wall, colorful wall hangings, objects on a shelf, a microphone on the table) within the child's sight that might elicit pointing gestures from the child. Note that all objects (except the CSBS DP materials in use at the moment) should be kept out of the child's reach during the Behavior Sample.

Seating Positions

During the warm-up, the child can be seated on the caregiver's lap, on the floor, or at a table. We recommend allowing the child to move around the room for the first several minutes. For the Behavior Sample, it is strongly recommended that the child be seated in a Sassy seat or a similar hanging seat that attaches to a sturdy table. If the child does not have adequate trunk support or this arrangement is not possible, the child can be seated in a high chair, a booster seat, or a child-size chair in a corner with a table positioned diagonally in front to limit the child's mobility. As an alternative, a child can be placed on a caregiver's lap, but periodic efforts should be made to have the child sit independently in order to maximize caregiver participation. The child may also be moved to the floor at any point between sampling contexts if he or she is becoming inattentive or fussy; however, it is best to move the child out of the seat only for a break and to put the child back in the seat for the remainder of the sample if at all possible.

During the CSBS DP Behavior Sample, the caregiver should be sitting to the child's right and the evaluator to the child's left, both equally distant from the child and within the child's visual field. It is recommended that the evaluator be positioned slightly in front of the child to enhance interaction. This arrangement can be accomplished by having the caregiver and child positioned on one side of the table and the evaluator on the adjacent side or by using a round table. Both adults should be sitting close enough to the child that the child can easily hand an object to them or touch them. Adjust the height of the seats so that the child can establish face-to-face contact with the adults with a predominantly horizontal but slightly upward gaze.

Keep all materials out of the child's sight and reach when they are not in use. To facilitate the sampling procedures, arrange materials in a container in the order of presentation (e.g., the kit carrying bag or a box). You may wish to separate the materials into two groups: 1) temptations and books and 2) symbolic and constructive play.

Sanitary and Safety Precautions

Any Behavior Sample evaluation materials a child can put in his or her mouth should be discarded or cleaned before being used with another child. Particular care should be taken when using the balloons. Do not allow the child to place more than the end of the balloon in his or her mouth. If the balloon breaks, all the pieces of the balloon should be disposed of immediately. The balloons should be discarded at the end of the session. Do not reuse the balloons. Any heavyweight 8-inch or 9-inch balloons can be purchased when the supply is exhausted. If a child is allergic to latex or if latex is not allowed in the clinical setting, substitute a nonlatex surgical glove, which can be inflated and deflated like a balloon. The baby bottles and nipples are genuine and can be sterilized in boiling water on a conventional stove or in a microwave oven. All other toys are washable and should be cleaned with antiseptic soap and water or alcohol wipes.

Table 5.1. Outline of sampling procedures and instructions

Warm-up

"We are going to begin by letting [child's name] get used to the room. You can hold him [her] on your lap or let him [her] play on the floor. We can use this time to go over the questionnaire."

Behavior sample

"We want to get a sample of how [child's name] communicates with sounds, gestures, or words. First, I am going to present some situations that will encourage [child's name] to communicate. Wait for [child's name] to communicate to you. Please try not to ask him [her] too many questions. When [child's name] does communicate, try to respond naturally, by helping him [her] or noticing what he [she] is playing with."

Opportunity 1
- Wind-up toy
- Toys in bag

Opportunity 2
- Balloon
- Toys in bag
- Gaze/point following probe

Opportunity 3
- Bubbles
- Toys in bag

Opportunity 4
- Jar
- Toys in bag

"Now we want to see what [child's name] does when looking at books. Try to avoid telling [child's name] what to look at or asking [child's name] to label the picture. Follow [child's name]'s lead by noticing or labeling the picture that he [she] directs your attention to."

Opportunity 5
- Books
- Gaze/point following probe

"Now we want to see how [child's name] plays with different sets of toys. Again, try to avoid telling [child's name] what to do or asking [child's name] questions. Follow [child's name]'s lead by commenting about what he [she] is doing."

Opportunity 6
- Symbolic play probe
  - Present feeding toy set
  - Provide verbal instructions and modeling
- Comprehension probe
  - Object names
  - Person names
  - Body parts
- Constructive play probe—Blocks

Note that the CSBS DP kit should not be used independently by children, even though many of the materials are ordinary children's toys. The child should never be left alone in the evaluation room and should not be allowed to play with the toys in the CSBS DP kit without careful adult supervision. With the exception of the balloon, most of the toys are safe for toddlers, but special care should be taken with infants. Young children should be allowed to explore the objects presented during the Behavior Sample but only with adult supervision. Exploration may include mouthing, but children should not be allowed to put entire objects in their mouths.

Sampling Contexts

It is highly desirable for the caregiver to participate actively during collection of the CSBS DP Behavior Sample. (However, it should be recognized that the Behavior

Sample is not designed to be a direct measure of caregiver–child interaction.) The instructions below are provided to encourage the caregiver to participate without being highly directive (i.e., excessive use of questions and commands). In the unlikely event that a caregiver should be unresponsive or ill at ease, the clinician should encourage caregiver participation. For the caregiver who is being too directive, the clinician should remind the parent to wait and follow the child's lead.

Procedures for each sampling context are described in depth below. Refer to Table 5.1 for an outline of the sampling procedures (these are also included on a laminated card in the forms packet). It is strongly recommended that the evaluator be familiar with the sampling and scoring procedures of the CSBS DP. Detailed scoring procedures appear on pages 46–62 of this manual. The CSBS DP tutorial videotapes should also be reviewed before attempting to administer the CSBS DP.

WARM-UP

The following instructions should be spoken to the caregiver before beginning:

"We are going to begin by letting [child's name] get used to the room. You can hold [child's name] on your lap or let him [her] play on the floor. We can use this time to go over the questionnaire."

The purpose of the warm-up is to allow the child and caregiver to settle in and become comfortable. The importance of the warm-up should not be underestimated. In our experience, an inadequate warm-up can be detrimental to the quality of the Behavior Sample. Minimal demands should be placed on the child during this time. The warm-up should last 2–10 minutes to allow time for the child to respond to the evaluator's solicitations for interactions. The child should be free to sit on the caregiver's lap or move around on the floor. During the warm-up, a few toys not included in the sampling procedures should be made available to the child. Select toys that are interesting to young children and that lend themselves to movement (e.g., push and ride vehicles, large balls, pop-up toys) as well as showing and turn taking (e.g., animal figures or blocks that can be taken in and out of a container, animal or person figures that fit in or ride on small vehicles). Each kit includes a toy for the warm-up, but other toys may also be available. Once the child is brought into the evaluation room, do not take time for the caregiver to complete the CSBS DP Caregiver Questionnaire before beginning the Behavior Sample because this action will interfere with the warm-up. As noted previously, the evaluator can use this time to ask questions about the child's medical and social history or clarify responses from the Caregiver Questionnaire. If video recording, make sure to begin running the camera during the warm-up to acclimate the adults and child to the movement of the light and noise from the camera.

While talking with the caregiver, the evaluator should occasionally offer items from the toy set to the child and attempt to engage the child in interaction. We have found that conversing informally with the caregiver initially without placing demands on the child allows both the caregiver and child to feel more comfortable. After a few minutes, try to engage the child affectively, by making the child laugh or smile, and vocally, by getting the child to make sounds or produce words. We have found that toys the child can sit on and roll or push may stimulate vocalizations. Begin the communicative temptations section when the child appears comfortable interacting with the evaluator; that is, when the child has smiled or laughed and vocalized (if able), or after 10 minutes. Keeping the warm-up to about 10 minutes will minimize child fatigue. If necessary, wait to finish taking the child's history or clarifying the questionnaire until all the sampling procedures are completed.

If the child remains hesitant to interact with the evaluator after the evaluator attempts to engage him or her, or if the child continually directs interactions toward the caregiver, simply instruct the caregiver to carry out each step of the sampling procedure as described below. We have found that younger children are more likely to direct more communication toward caregivers than unfamiliar adults.

BEHAVIOR SAMPLING PROCEDURES

Present the following six sampling opportunities for the child to display communicative and symbolic behaviors. Provide the following instructions to the caregiver before beginning:

"We want to get a sample of how [child's name] communicates with sounds, gestures, or words. First, I am going to present some situations that will encourage [child's name] to communicate. Wait for [child's name] to communicate to you. Please try not to ask him [her] too many questions. When [child's name] does communicate, try to respond naturally, by helping him [her] or noticing what he [she] is playing with."

The first four sampling opportunities are communicative temptations that provide opportunities for the child to request help; however, the child may protest or comment on the event. The evaluator and caregiver should respond naturally to the child's communicative intent by, for example, removing the object protested or commenting about the object referenced.

Communicative temptations should be presented in the order listed next. Each temptation is followed by a scoring opportunity during which the child plays with a toy. About 1–2 minutes should be spent on each temptation and about 30 seconds on each scoring opportunity in order to get through the temptations in 5–10 minutes. The purpose is to get a sample of the child's range of communicative behaviors in a brief amount of time rather than multiple examples of each behavior. Everything needed for the communicative temptations is included in the CSBS DP kit except the food for the jar temptation (Sampling Opportunity 4).

When first presenting each temptation, wait and look expectantly at the child. If the child does not readily initiate a communicative act, encourage the child by using the following prompts, as needed, in the order listed:

1. Say, "Need help?" with a rising intonation.

2. Extend an open hand on the table, at least 12 inches from the object.
3. Move the open hand to within 3 inches of the object, but do not touch it.
4. Repeat the temptation from the beginning.

The evaluator should wait about 7 seconds (counting silently "one thousand one, one thousand two...one thousand seven") after each prompt before presenting the next one. If the child fusses, protests, or shows no interest in a temptation, move on to the next one and return to that temptation if time allows.

SAMPLING OPPORTUNITY 1: WIND-UP TOY

Choose one of the two wind-up toys included in the CSBS DP kit.

- Activate a wind-up toy, and then let it deactivate. Allow the child to pick it up, and wait for the child to signal for your help. If the child does not pick it up within about 10 seconds, give it to the child and wait.
- After the child's *first* communicative signal to request, reactivate the wind-up toy. Let it deactivate. Allow the child to pick it up, or hand it to the child and wait for the child to signal for your help.
- After the child's *second* communicative signal to request, activate the wind-up toy, and then remove it from the table, while saying, "Bye-bye (name of animal)."

Scoring Opportunity 1

While the child is engaged with the wind-up toy, score the occurrence of as many behaviors displayed by the child as possible on the Behavior Sample: Scoring Worksheet under the column for *Sampling Opportunity 1: Wind-Up Toy* for the Communication Scales, which are the first 15 scales. After putting away the wind-up toy, present the toys in the bag.

Toys in the Bag

Use the cloth bag and four toys: the two teethers and the two animal figures. Either ahead of time or out of the child's sight, put all four toys into the bag.

- Shake the cloth bag containing the four toys to attract the child's attention. Place the bag in front of the child and encourage the child to take one of the toys out of the bag. If the child does not take a toy, hand one of the toys to the child and allow the child to examine the toy. Then, remove the bag, which now contains the three remaining toys, but allow the child to hold the first toy or set it aside.
- While the child is exploring the first object from the bag, score the occurrence of the remaining communicative behaviors that occurred during Sampling

Opportunity 1. If the child displays pertinent communicative behaviors that can be scored while exploring the toy from the bag, credit the child for those behaviors with the previous opportunity. Make sure to score all 15 communicative behaviors before presenting the next opportunity. If the child is not interested in the toy from the bag, ask the caregiver to engage the child for a moment or offer the child a preferred toy from the warm-up.

SAMPLING OPPORTUNITY 2: BALLOON

Use two balloons of the same color, one for you to blow and one for the child.

- Blow up your balloon. Hold the balloon with some air in it near the child, and encourage the child to touch or squeeze the balloon. Let it deflate slowly, pointing escaping air away from the child. *(For very young or cautious children, take particular care to let the air out slowly and quietly to prevent scaring the child.)* Hand the child's balloon to the child while holding onto your balloon, and wait for the child to signal for your help.
- After the child's *first* communicative signal to request, take back the child's balloon but blow up your balloon again, and let it deflate. Hand the child's balloon back to the child, and wait for the child to signal for your help.
- After the child's *second* communicative signal to request, blow up the balloon. Let it deflate, and then remove it from the table, while saying, "Bye-bye balloon."

Scoring Opportunity 2

While the child is engaged with the balloon, score the occurrence of as many behaviors displayed by the child as possible on the Behavior Sample: Scoring Worksheet under the column for *Sampling Opportunity 2: Balloon* for the Communication Scales. After putting away the balloon, present the toys in the bag that now contains three toys, following the instructions described previously. Use this time to score the occurrence of all remaining communicative behaviors that occurred during Sampling and Scoring Opportunity 2.

Gaze/Point Following Probe

When you are done scoring but before putting away the toy from the bag, ask the caregiver to engage the child with the toy. Call the child's name to get the child's attention and say, "Look," while pointing and looking at an object or picture at a distance on the wall or on a shelf behind the child and over his or her left shoulder (i.e., the same side that the evaluator is sitting). If 0° is the point directly in front of the child and 180° is directly behind the child, the evaluator should be sitting at about 45°, and the object or picture should be placed at about 135°, so that the child is following a change of less than 90° visual angle. Try to get the child to look in the direction you are pointing.

SAMPLING OPPORTUNITY 3: BUBBLES

Use the jar of bubbles.

- Open the jar of bubbles, and blow a few up in the air away from the child's face. Catch one bubble on the wand, and encourage the child to pop it. Close the jar of bubbles tightly, and hand the jar to the child. Wait for the child to signal for your help.
- After the child's *first* communicative signal to request, open the jar, blow a few bubbles, and again catch one on the wand. Close the jar of bubbles tightly, hand it to the child, and wait for the child to signal for your help.
- After the child's *second* communicative signal to request, open the jar, blow a few bubbles, and then remove the jar from the table, while saying, "Bye-bye, bubbles."

Scoring Opportunity 3

While the child is engaged with the bubbles, score the occurrence of as many behaviors displayed by the child as possible on the Behavior Sample: Scoring Worksheet under the column for *Sampling Opportunity 3: Bubbles* for the Communication Scales. After putting away the bubbles, present the toys in the bag that now contains two toys (do not bring out a toy that you have already used with the child). Follow the instructions described previously. Use this time to score the occurrence of all remaining communicative behaviors that occurred during Sampling and Scoring Opportunity 3.

SAMPLING OPPORTUNITY 4: JAR

Use the jar with a lid and Cheerios (or a substitute). Before beginning this temptation, ask the caregiver if it is okay for the child to eat the Cheerios. If it is not, substitute an acceptable food or small toy that will fit in the jar.

- Put one Cheerio (or other desired food or toy item that will fit in the jar) on the table in front of the child and encourage the child to take it and eat it (or examine the toy) to establish interest. Then, put a small handful of Cheerios in the jar while the child is watching. Close the jar, shake the Cheerios around to attract the child's attention, and then put the jar on the table within the child's reach. Wait for the child to signal for your help.
- After the child's *first* communicative signal to request, open the jar and put one Cheerio on the table for the child to take, close the jar, and put the jar on the table in front of the child. Wait for the child to signal for your help.
- After the child's *second* communicative signal to request, open the jar and put one Cheerio on the table for the child to take, then remove the jar from the table while saying, "Bye-bye, Cheerios."

Scoring Opportunity 4

While the child is eating the food in the jar (or examining the toy), score the occurrence of as many behaviors displayed by the child as possible on the Behavior Sample: Scoring Worksheet under the column for *Sampling Opportunity 4: Jar* for the Communication Scales. After putting away the jar, present the toys in the bag that now contains one toy, following the instructions described previously. Use this time to score the occurrence of all remaining communicative behaviors that occurred during Sampling and Scoring Opportunity 4.

SAMPLING OPPORTUNITY 5: BOOKS

Give the following instructions to the caregiver before presenting the books.

"Now we want to see what [child's name] does when looking at books. Try to avoid telling [child's name] what to look at or asking [child's name] to label the picture. Follow [child's name] lead by noticing or labeling the picture that he [she] directs your attention to."

Use the three books.

- Show the child three books and encourage him or her to select one. Remove the books that the child does not select. Allow the child to examine the chosen book while the evaluator displays interest in it. The evaluator should respond naturally to the child's communicative behaviors by acknowledging, commenting on, or expanding on what the child is looking at, pointing at, or communicating about in the book. Avoid giving the child commands or asking the child questions except to request clarification or further information.

- If the child looks through the first book very quickly, offer the child the remaining two books and encourage him or her to select one. Remove the other book and allow the child to examine the chosen book as described previously. After the child looks through the book, remove it.

Scoring Opportunity 5

Present the child with the remaining book or books and encourage him or her to take it or select one. Encourage the caregiver and child to engage with the book. Use this time to score the occurrence of communicative behaviors during *Sampling Opportunity 5: Books* for the Communication Scales. If the child displays pertinent communicative behaviors while exploring the last book, credit the child for those behaviors with the previous opportunity.

Gaze/Point Following Probe

When you are done scoring, but before you put away the book, have the caregiver continue to engage the child with the book. Call the child by name and say, "Look," while pointing to an object at a distance on the wall or shelf across midline to the child's right (i.e., the opposite side that the evaluator is sitting). If 0° is the point directly in front of the child and 180° is directly behind the child, the evaluator should be sitting at about 45°, and the object or picture should be placed at about 270° (i.e., 90° to the child's right), so that the child is following a change of more than a 90° visual angle. Try to get the child to look in the direction you are pointing.

SAMPLING OPPORTUNITY 6: PLAY

Sampling Opportunity 6 consists of three parts to probe symbolic play, comprehension, and constructive play. Give the following instructions to the caregiver before presenting the play materials.

"Now we want to see how [child's name] plays with different sets of toys. Again try to avoid telling [child's name] what to do or asking [child's name] questions. Follow [child's name] lead by commenting about what he [she] is doing."

Symbolic Play Probe

Use the plush doll character (Big Bird is used in the CSBS DP Videotape Tutorial) and symbolic play feeding toy set, which consists of two cups, two bowls, two spoons, two bottles, one frying pan and lid, one spatula, one mixing bowl, and one serving spoon.

- Give the child the plush doll. Then, give the child the following four objects from the feeding toy set: the cup, the bowl, the spoon, and the bottle. Bring out the matching four objects, keep two and give two to the caregiver. Respond naturally to the child's play and communicative behaviors by acknowledging, commenting on, or expanding on the child's communication and by imitating the child's actions on objects. Encourage the caregiver to imitate the child's actions with the two objects. Avoid giving the child commands or asking the child questions except to request clarification or further information.
- When the child has examined the first four objects and used at least one object functionally toward self or others, bring out the remaining objects, which include the frying pan and lid, spatula, mixing bowl, and serving spoon, and allow the child to initiate play for a few minutes with these toys. For very young children who are primarily mouthing, banging, and dropping the objects, you should skip bringing out the remaining objects.
- During the play sample, if the child is not demonstrating action schemes toward other, direct the child's attention to the caregiver or the plush doll by the using gestures or a simple statement, such as, "Oh, look at Big Bird. He's hungry."

- After the child initiates play with the feeding toy set for a few minutes, probe for the use of more sophisticated symbolic play, first by giving verbal instructions (e.g., "Big Bird is hungry," "Show me how you feed Big Bird," "Show me how you make Big Bird's food"). Then, model the use of more sophisticated play with one utensil, allow the child to take a turn using the same utensil, and encourage the child to demonstrate the action scheme with a different utensil without modeling. For example, if the child fed the plush doll but did not sequence actions, model stirring and feeding the plush doll with the spoon.

Because the child can be credited for imitation of an action scheme but must use an imitated action scheme twice, it is important for the evaluator and caregiver to model action schemes enough but not too much. Allow the child to use each object spontaneously first, and imitate what the child is doing but make sure to model at a level higher than the child is displaying in regard to three dimensions: the variety of functional use of objects, the orientation of actions toward others, and the sequence of actions. Allow the child to take a few turns with the objects before modeling again.

Comprehension Probe

For the comprehension probe, it is essential that no gestural or other cues be given that may guide the child's responses to assure that linguistic comprehension is being measured.

- After the child finishes playing with the feeding toy set, say "Time to pick up," and begin removing some of the objects, but leave the cup, the bowl, the spoon, the bottle, and two additional objects as foils. Ask the child to give you each object by name. Say, "Give me the _____ (e.g., cup, bowl, spoon, bottle)," while extending one hand out with the palm up to receive the object. A correct response is the child touching or giving the object named. You should applaud and praise the child for giving you an object. You may repeat each object name once; however, do not repeat the name if the child is identifying the wrong object. Remove each object as the child gives it to you, making sure there are at least three choices of objects for the last trial. If the child begins removing objects before you present the name, put the objects back on the table and instruct the child to "wait" (use a palm toward child gesture) and "listen" (use a pointing gesture to your ears). You may present up to four different names of objects; stop when the child has correctly identified three different objects.

It is often difficult to get a young child to attend to and comply with a verbal instruction, and, therefore, an attempt at a trial may be "botched." An example of a botched trial is if the child begins to pick up a spoon just as you say the word *spoon* because you don't know whether the child responded to your instruction or just wanted to hold the spoon. Another example of a botched trial is if you or the parent inadvertently point to the object while you name it. While a botched trial should be readministered, care should be taken not to present more than eight trials (i.e., eight trials that are not botched)—at the most, four object names each repeated once. If the child misses two object names in a row, you may discontinue object names.

- Next, ask the child to identify person names, using the choices of the caregiver(s), the child, and the stuffed plush doll (e.g., Big Bird). Say, "Where is Mommy?" Again, other carrier phrases may be used and additional cues should not be provided. A correct response is the child touching or showing the agent named or making a clear change in direction of gaze to the agent. You should applaud and praise the child for identifying the person or agent. You may repeat each person's name once; however, do not repeat the name if the child is identifying the wrong agent. You may present all three agents; stop when the child has correctly identified two different agents. If the child misses two person names in a row, you may discontinue person names.

- Next, ask the child to identify different body parts. Select body parts from the following choices, beginning with the ones the caregiver indicated the child knows: head, hair, eyes, nose, mouth, ears, tummy, hand, and feet. Even if the caregiver says that the child does not know any body parts, still attempt to follow the procedures. Tell the caregiver that it is informative to try. For example, say, "Where is Katie's mouth?" Give stress to the lexical items being tested. Other carrier phrases may be used: "Point to ______" or "Show me ______." The child can identify the body part on him- or herself, on the caregiver, on the evaluator, or on the plush doll. A correct response is the child's touching or showing the body part named or making a clear change in direction of gaze to that body part. You should applaud and praise the child for identifying a body part. You may repeat the name of each body part once to get the child to identify it, but do not repeat the name if the child is identifying the wrong body part. You may present up to four different body parts. Stop when the child has correctly identified three different body parts. If the child misses two body parts in a row, you may discontinue body parts.

Constructive Play Probe

Use the five blocks.

- Engage the child in a turn-taking game of building a tower and knocking it down. Then, give the child an opportunity to build a tower without assistance. If the child does not readily build a tower, hand the child one block at a time, and encourage the child to build. Applaud and praise the child for attempting to stack the blocks.

Scoring Opportunity 6

While the child is engaged with the play materials from the symbolic play probe through blocks, score the occurrence of communicative behaviors on the Behavior Sample: Scoring Worksheet for *Sampling Opportunity 6: Play* for the Communication Scales. While the child is using the symbolic play materials, score the use of action schemes displayed by the child on the Behavior Sample: Scoring Worksheet for the first three Symbolic Behavior Scales under *Object Use* (Scales 17–19). Once scoring for these items is complete, proceed to the comprehension probe (Scale 16), and then score that item. While the child is engaged with the blocks, score the child's performance on the Behavior Sample: Scoring Worksheet for *Stacks tower of blocks* (Scale 20).

CSBS DP CAREGIVER PERCEPTION RATING

Immediately following the sample, the caregiver should be asked to complete the CSBS DP Behavior Sample: Caregiver Perception Rating. On this form, the caregiver rates the child's behavior during the sample in terms of how typical it was. An alternative is to interview the caregiver using this form. The Behavior Sample: Caregiver Perception Rating informs the evaluator about the representativeness of the sample. Therefore, if the caregiver notes that his or her child's behavior was less than typical, particularly on the level of communication (#6) and play behavior (#7), contrast the child's behavior during the sample with the information reported in the CSBS DP Caregiver Questionnaire. You may need to consider obtaining another sample and/or observing the child in a different context. Report any discrepancies when interpreting results.

TIPS FOR PUTTING CAREGIVERS AT EASE

It is natural for caregivers to be cautious or uncomfortable in a testing situation because they are unsure of what you are asking their child to do or what they should do, and they want their child to perform at his or her best. The following are some strategies that we have found helpful to put caregivers at ease and to encourage their participation.

- During the warm-up, give the caregiver an idea of what you will be doing with him or her and his or her child and how long it will take. For example, say "We are going to be playing with toys. You will be in the room with your child the whole time. We will be done in about 30 minutes."
- Give clear instructions so that the caregiver understands what should be done.
- Make sure the caregiver is sitting close to the child and is within the child's reach.
- During the sample, give the caregiver an idea of how much time is left. At the end of the temptations, let the caregiver know that you are about halfway done. At the end of the symbolic play, let the caregiver know that you have only a few quick things left.
- Tell the caregiver something positive about how the child is doing, such as, "See how (child's name) asks for help by giving you the object" or, "He is so expressive with his eyes that he lets me know what he's interested in by looking at it."
- Give the caregiver an idea about the kinds of behaviors you are measuring. For example, say, "We are interested in how your child uses eye gaze, facial expressions, and gestures to communicate."
- Tell the caregiver something positive about how they are doing. For example, say, "You are doing great at waiting and responding to (child's name) attempts to communicate" or, "It is great the way you are naming the pictures that (child's name) is pointing to."

- Make sure to encourage the caregiver to interact with the child. While the instructions are one way to do this, there are also several other ways. Tell the child to give the object to the caregiver to get help or to share it with the caregiver. For example, if the child gives the wind-up toy to you, when the child has the balloon, say, "Ask mommy to help blow," while pointing to the caregiver. During the scoring opportunities, make an effort to stay out of the interaction by focusing your attention on the worksheet to give the caregiver a chance to take the lead. Make sure to give the caregiver one of the books, and ask the caregiver to share the book with the child. Make sure to invite the caregiver to play with the child using the matching symbolic play objects.

TIPS FOR GETTING THE MOST COMMUNICATION FROM VERY YOUNG CHILDREN

- Make sure to give the child ample time to get comfortable during the warm-up and to get the child to vocalize and to display positive affect before you begin the sample. We have found that movement is the key to both vocalizations and affect.
- Make sure to allow and encourage the child to initiate during the sample by waiting and looking expectantly at the child.
- Use exaggerated facial expression and intonation to capture the child's attention and encourage affect and vocalization. For example, as the child pulls the first object out of the bag, use a surprise/delight facial expression and say, "Oh, you found Big Bird!" with an exaggerated intonation contour to stress "Big Bird."
- Be overly responsive to joint attention. It is easy to notice if the child is requesting help or protesting. Make sure also to notice when the child is drawing your attention to something by looking at it and commenting about it. For example, if the child shows you an object or points to something, make sure to focus your attention on that object and label it or comment about it. If the child is not using gestures or sounds to direct your attention to objects, comment on what the child is looking at. Be particularly attentive when the child shifts gaze between you and an object. You can notice an object by looking at it attentively and using a general exclamation like "ooo," by labeling the object, or by describing an action or attribute of the object.
- If the child communicates about something other than the CSBS DP materials during the sample or about CSBS DP materials that you have removed, make sure to respond. For example, if you are offering the child books, and the child reaches toward the bag to request more Cheerios, then bring the Cheerios back and give the child one more or tell the child he or she can have more in a little while.
- Remember that if the child fusses or protests, he or she is communicating. Don't panic. Make every effort to help calm down the child, but don't overreact. Ask the caregiver for ideas on how to calm the child. Learning how easily a child calms down and what helps to calm the child is important information for communication development. Young children will often calm down quickly if the adults around them are responsive but not overreactive. Distracting the child with a new or desired object is often all that is needed.

- If the child's affect is very flat, make an extra effort to get the child to laugh. Most children like getting tickled in the game of "I'm gonna get you." Play this game with one of the objects that the child pulls out of the bag in an effort to get the child to laugh.
- Be very familiar with the sampling procedures. Make sure to practice the procedures so that you are very comfortable with all the steps and materials. As the procedures become more automatic, you can focus your attention on putting the caregiver at ease and being responsive to the child.
- Be very familiar with the scoring procedures. Understanding what behaviors you are measuring in the sample will greatly enhance your ability to offer support and be responsive to the child during the sample.

SCORING PROCEDURES FOR THE BEHAVIOR SAMPLE

The Behavior Sample for the CSBS DP is designed to produce a record of the interactions between a parent, a young child, and an evaluator. This sample may be scored in one of two ways: in-vivo (i.e., during the sample) or later if the sample is recorded on videotape. In either case, the CSBS DP Behavior Sample: Scoring Worksheet must be completed. The results should be scored and reported on the CSBS DP Behavior Sample: Scoring Summary.

The CSBS DP Behavior Sample is divided into six sampling opportunities: wind-up toy, balloon, bubbles, jar, books, and play. Each sampling opportunity begins with the initiation of that context and ends with the initiation of the next context. Any behaviors displayed during the scoring opportunity (i.e., the toys in the bag) or in between sampling opportunities should be scored with the previous sampling opportunity. The play sampling opportunity includes both symbolic play and blocks and ends after the blocks.

The evaluator should enter a √ or a + during each sampling opportunity to indicate the presence of the child's behavior or should leave it blank to indicate the absence. First, you should decide whether the child displayed a particular communicative or symbolic behavior and record this information in the appropriate space. For example, during the first scoring opportunity, begin by judging the child's use of alternating eye gaze. You will need to make a quick decision about whether the child displayed each behavior during the first scoring opportunity. You should work quickly down the column recording judgments about each scale. If you are completing the worksheet while viewing a videotape of the sample, the videotape can be paused briefly at the end of each sampling opportunity.

The Communication Scales (Scales 1–15; see Table 2.1) are sampled during all six sampling opportunities of the entire CSBS DP Behavior Sample. That is, the Communication Scales are evaluated from the wind-up toy through the blocks. Communication Scales 4–15 measure different parameters of the child's use of communicative acts (which are defined next). Scales 1–3 measure Emotion and Eye Gaze, which may or may not occur along with a communicative act. The Symbolic Behavior Scales (Scales 16–20) are evaluated during Sampling Opportunity 6, which is designed to probe these behaviors.

Definitions of the 20 scales are provided next, followed by detailed instructions for completing the CSBS DP Behavior Sample: Scoring Worksheet.

For a behavior to be considered a communicative act, the answer to all three of the following questions must be yes; that is, the behavior must be described by at least one of the options under each question.

1. Was the act a gesture, vocalization, or verbalization?
   ___ Giving object to adult
   ___ Touching adult's hand, arm, body, or face
   ___ Moving adult's hand or face
   ___ Moving object toward or away from adult
   ___ Head shaking or nodding
   ___ Hitting, biting, or pinching self or adult
   ___ Throwing or dropping objects
   ___ Showing off without object
   ___ Showing off with object near child's face
   ___ Making indicative gesture
   ___ Pointing with finger or fingers (not palm)
   ___ Tapping with finger or fingers (not palm)
   ___ Raising arms
   ___ Open-hand reaching with minimal body movement
   ___ Showing object (holding object up toward adult in reference to child's midline and not releasing object)
   ___ Making depictive gesture (i.e., pantomine-like actions)
   ___ Waving
   ___ Clapping
   ___ Nontranscribable vocalizations
   ___ Transcribable vocalizations
   ___ Verbalization (single or multiword utterances)
2. Was the act directed toward the adult?
   ___ Giving object to adult
   ___ Touching adult
   ___ Moving object or palm-up reach toward or away from adult in reference to the child's midline
   ___ Using any other gesture and looking at adult
   ___ Using any other gesture and a vocalization/verbalization
   ___ Using a vocalization/verbalization and looking at adult
3. Was the act used as a communicative signal to serve a communicative function?
   ___ Regulating adult's behavior to do something or to stop doing something (behavior regulation)
   ___ Attracting adult's attention to look at or notice self (social interaction)
   ___ Directing adult's attention to look at or notice an object or event (joint attention)
   ___ Unclear communicative function (unclear if act serves function of behavior regulation, social interaction, or joint attention)

Figure 5.2. Decision making for identifying communicative acts.

DEFINITIONS FOR THE COMMUNICATION AND SYMBOLIC SCALES

A communicative act is the primary unit of analysis for Scales 4–15. Therefore, the first step in learning how to rate the communicative behaviors is to identify a communicative act. A *communicative act* is defined as an interactive behavior that consists of a gesture, vocalization, or verbalization that is directed toward the adult and that serves a communicative function. Rules for decision making about identifying communicative acts are listed in Figure 5.2, and are based on the CSBS (Wetherby & Prizant, 1993).

Only behaviors included in the list of gestures in Figure 5.2 and speech and non-speech vocalizations may be considered communicative acts. In addition, only those gestures, vocalizations, or verbalizations directed toward the adult that serve a communicative function (as indicated in Figure 5.2) are to be included as communicative acts. Keep in mind that parameters assessed on Scales 4–15 pertain only to behaviors meeting criteria for communicative acts. Remember that eye gaze alone is not a communicative act and that behaviors, such as taking an object or reaching to take, are not counted. Gestures such as a reach or point are only counted if they are directed to an adult and used as a communicative signal. Similarly, vocalizations or words are only counted if they are directed to an adult either with eye gaze or gestures. Directing a communicative act to an adult with eye gaze means looking at an adult immediately before, during, or after the act and does not require a three-point gaze shift.

For the communicative temptations, the topic is determined by the particular objects and/or actions being used. For the books, the topic is limited to what is portrayed on two facing pages. A new topic begins when a page is turned. Thus, a child may produce more than one communicative act about two facing pages if there is a pause greater than 3 seconds or if the adult takes one or more turns involving speech or conventional gestures. Incomplete acts may occur if the child abandons a communicative act or is interrupted before completion. Incomplete acts should not be rated. Complete acts displayed by the child should be counted even if an adult does not respond to the communicative attempt.

COMMUNICATION SCALES

Emotion and Eye Gaze

Communicative development and interactions are rooted in early social and affective development in infants. Eye gaze and the expression of emotion are signals that guide the caregiver's responses to the infant and regulate social interactions. Scales 1–3 measure the child's expression of emotion and use of eye gaze during the first six sampling opportunities. For these three scales, eye gaze and facial expression may be part of a communicative act, as defined previously and used in Scales 4–15, but may also occur without a communicative act. Therefore, credit may be given for parameters of a communicative act (i.e., use of communication, gestures, sounds, and words) and emotion and eye gaze (i.e., gaze shift, positive affect, gaze following) when they occur simultaneously. Unlike Scales 4–15, these three scales can provide useful information about children who demonstrate few or no communicative acts.

Scale 1 is a measure of the child's use of gaze shifts for social referencing during interactions. A *gaze shift* is defined as alternating eye gaze between a person and an object and back. Eye gaze must be directed to an adult's face; gaze directed to any other part of the body (e.g., hands) is not credited. Thus, one gaze shift (called a *three-point gaze shift*) may be either a person–object–person gaze shift (i.e., when the child is looking at a person, shifts gaze to an object, and then immediately shifts back to the person) or an object–person–object gaze shift (i.e., when the child is looking at an object, shifts gaze to a person, and then immediately shifts back to the object). Furthermore, another gaze shift (called a *four-point gaze shift*) may also be an object–person A–person B–object gaze shift (i.e., when the child is looking at an object, shifts gaze to person A, immediately shifts gaze to person B, and then shifts back to the object). A gaze shift may occur without a communicative act or may support a communicative act.

Scale 2 is a measure of sociability or sharing of positive affective states. A display of positive affect is a *clear* facial expression of pleasure or excitement, which may or may not be accompanied by a vocalization (e.g., laughter, squeal). Because communication development is rooted in sharing affect, this scale measures the display of positive affect that is directed to an adult. Do not count subtle or ambiguous affective displays. Shared positive affect is measured by counting the display of positive affect coordinated with gaze directed toward the adult, immediately before, during, or after the affect display. An instance of positive affect is terminated when a child shifts to a neutral or negative state. The display of positive affect with directed gaze should be counted, but displays of positive affect without directed gaze toward the adult are not counted. Note that a gaze shift is not necessary. If the directed gaze involves a three- or four-point gaze shift, then the child can receive credit for both positive affect and gaze shift.

Scale 3 is a measure of gaze/point following. This is a child's ability to follow the visual regard of another person's gaze and point at a distance. Two probes to measure gaze following are presented at the end of Sampling Opportunity 2 and 5, which were adapted from Mundy et al. (1995). Gaze/point following is credited when the child turns his or her head at least 45° and directs gaze where the evaluator is pointing.

Communication

Scales 4–7 are a measure of the rate and function of communication. Scale 4 is a measure of the rate of communicating. Rate of communicating with gestures and/or vocalizations in typically developing children increased substantially from an average of about one act per minute for 1-year-olds at the prelinguistic stage to about five acts per minute for 2-year-olds at the multiword stage (Wetherby et al., 1988; Wetherby, Yonclas, & Bryan, 1989). Thus, rate of communicating is a useful index of communication development for children who have no or few intelligible words. Using the CSBS definition of a communicative act, the number of communicative acts should be considered from the beginning of each sampling opportunity. Rate of communicating is sampled by documenting the number of communicative acts up to three per sampling opportunity. Record whether the child displays zero, one, two, or at least three communicative acts during the sampling opportunity. Each sampling opportunity has turns structured so that the child may readily initiate at least three communicative acts (e.g., two during each communicative temptation and one during the toys in the bag).

Scales 5, 6, and 7 measure the communicative functions (i.e., the purposes served by communicative acts) that the child uses in each of the major categories of behavioral regulation, social interaction, and joint attention. A categorical framework for communicative functions used by young children is defined in depth in Table 5.2. The earliest emerging functions that are used by children younger than 12 months of age are behavior regulation (e.g., request for object/action, protest)

Table 5.2. Definitions of categories of communicative functions

Behavior regulation—acts used to regulate the behavior of another person to obtain a specific result. The child's goal is to get the adult to do something or stop doing something.

Request object/action—acts used to direct another to give a desired object or to carry out an action

Protest object/action—acts used to refuse an object that is not desired or to direct another to cease an action that is not desired

Social interaction—acts used to attract or maintain another's attention to oneself. The child's goal is to get the adult to look at/notice him or her.

Request social routine—acts used to direct another to begin or continue carrying out a game-like social interaction

Request comfort—acts used to seek another's attention to comfort from wariness, distress, or frustration

Call—acts used to gain the attention of another to indicate that a communicative act is to follow

Greet—acts used to indicate notice of a person or object's presence, or to signal the initiation or termination of an interaction

Show off—acts used to attract another's attention to oneself by displaying a performance

Request permission—acts used to seek another's consent to carry out an action; involves carrying out or wanting to carry out the action

Joint attention—acts used to direct another's attention to an object, event, or topic of a communicative act. The child's goal is to get the adult to look at or notice something.

Comment on object/action—acts used to direct another's attention to an entity or event

Request information—acts used to seek information, explanations, or clarifications about an entity, event, or previous utterance; includes wh-questions and other utterances with a rising intonation contour

Unclear—acts used for a communicative purpose but there is insufficient information to determine which functional category is most appropriate. It cannot be determined whether child's goal is to get adult to do something/stop doing something, to attend to him/her, or to attend to something.

Sources: Bruner (1981); Coggins & Carpenter (1981); Seibert, Hogan, & Mundy (1982); Wetherby et al. (1988); Wetherby & Prutting (1984); and Wetherby & Prizant (1993).

and social interaction (e.g., request social routine, request comfort, calling, greeting, showing off). Joint attention should be emerging at about 12 months of age. The most frequent communicative functions used by children 18 to 24 months of age are behavior regulation (i.e., request object/action) and joint attention (i.e., comment on object/action). It is important to consider the communicative function separate from communicative means because a specific means can serve different functions. For example, a pointing gesture may be used for behavior regulation (e.g., request object) or for joint attention (e.g., comment). Similarly, a giving gesture is usually used for behavior regulation (e.g., request action) but may also be used to establish joint attention (e.g., comment). The interactive context needs to be referred to in determining function.

For Scales 5, 6, and 7, it is important to recognize and distinguish among the child's attempts to 1) get an adult to do something or stop doing something with an object (behavior regulation), 2) draw an adult's attention to self (social interaction), and 3) get the adult to look at or notice an object or event but not do something to it (joint attention). Judgments about communicative function are inferred from the context based on the child's communicative goal or purpose. The child's use of at least one communicative act for behavior regulation during each sampling opportunity should be recorded for Scale 5. One communicative act should be scored for social interaction for Scale 6, and one communicative act for joint attention for Scale 7 during each sampling opportunity.

Gestures

Communicative means are behaviors used to express communicative intentions. Scales 8 and 9 focus on the quality of gestures or gestural means used to communicate, either without vocalizations or in coordination with vocal acts. A *gesture* is defined as a nonvocal behavior directed to another person that serves a communicative function. A gesture typically involves movement of the hand or head. Directed eye gaze without hand or head movement does not count as a gesture. Specific examples of communicative gestures are listed in Figure 5.2. Holding, touching, or taking an object does not count as a gesture unless the child is directing the gesture toward the adult (e.g., showing, giving), as delineated in Figure 5.2.

Scale 8 is a measure of the variety of conventional gestures. For this scale, conventional gestures include the following eight gestures: gives, shows, pushes/pulls away, reaches, points, waves, nodds head, and shakes head. Reaching includes open-hand reaching using one hand with the palm up or down and reaching with both arms (e.g., raising arms). To be credited as using one of these eight conventional gestures, a child must display at least one communicative act involving that gesture. Research has demonstrated that typically developing children use a variety of conventional gestures during the prelinguistic stage and that they are precursors to the emergence of words (Bates et al., 1987). The inventory of different conventional gestures displayed should be recorded.

Scale 9 is a measure of the sophistication of hand gestures from contact to distal. This scale addresses only a subset of gestures—those involving hand movement. A contact gesture is made when the child's hand actually touches another person or object. Examples include manipulating the adult's hand, giving an object, showing an object, and touching or tapping on an object or picture while pointing. A distal gesture is made when the child's hand does not touch a person or object while gesturing. Examples include using an open-handed reach, pointing at a distance, and waving. Both contact and distal gestures may be conventional gestures but are not restricted to only conventional gestures, as defined in Scale 7. For example, a child may use a depictive gesture without touching an object or person to request opening the jar. This would be counted as a distal gesture but not a conventional gesture. The child's use of a distal gesture during each sampling opportunity should be recorded.

Sounds

Scales 10 and 11 address communicative acts that meet the criteria in Figure 5.2 and consist of or include a vocalization. For these scales, only transcribeable vowel or consonant-like sounds are considered vocalizations. Nontranscribeable sounds such as laughs, cries, sighs, lip smacks, trills, and raspberries should not be included in this rating. A vocalization *must include a vowel sound* and may also include a consonant that precedes or follows the vowel. For example, a whine produced with the mouth closed approximating /m/ would not contain a vowel and thus would not be counted. (Nontranscribable sounds may be rated as communicative acts for Scales 4–9 if they are directed toward the adult with a gesture or eye gaze and serve a communicative function, as defined in Figure 5.2.) Thus, Scales 10 and 11 address only a subset of vocal acts, those that are transcribable sounds and include a vowel sound. It is important to keep in mind that vocal acts scored for Scales 10 and 11 can be either recognizable words or transcribable sounds that are not recognizable words. In addition, vocal acts can be produced either spontaneously or imitatively.

Scales 10 and 11 are designed to assess the composition of consonant and vowel sounds within syllables in communicative acts that contain a transcribable vocalization. Scale 10 rates the use of syllables containing consonants, and Scale 11 rates the inventory of different consonants.

For Scales 10 and 11, the consonants of particular interest are the ones that emerge earliest. To simplify evaluation judgments, we have included the 10 consonants that are most likely to be used by children 2 years of age and younger. Consonants other than these 10 should not be recorded. It should be noted that the *H* and glottal stop are generally not considered consonants for young children and should not be included. (A glottal stop is closure of the vocal folds that stops the flow of air, as between the vowels in "uh oh.") In addition, young children do not yet consistently distinguish between voiced and voiceless cognates (e.g., /ba/ versus /pa/) in their productions. Therefore, productions that sound like /pa/, /ta/, or /ka/ should be credited as /ba/, /da/, or /ga/, respectively. Table 5.3 lists transcribable consonants that should be considered in rating Scales 10 and 11.

Scale 10 assesses the child's use of syllables containing at least one consonant in vocal communicative acts. The communicative act does not need to include a recognizable word. In considering syllables with consonants, the consonant may precede or follow a vowel. The child's use of a syllable containing a consonant should be credited for each sampling opportunity. In contrast to Scale 11, for Scale 10 the variety of consonants should not influence the rating; that is, the child may use the same consonant in all syllables and be credited once for each sampling opportunity.

Scale 11 is a measure of the variety of different consonants used by the child within vocal communicative acts. On Scale 11, the child needs to use a consonant only once to be credited for it. Remember, the vocal act does not need to be a recognizable word. The different consonants the child uses in vocal acts during any of the six sampling opportunities should be recorded on the checklist of consonants.

Words

For Scales 12–15, a *word* or *lexical form* is defined as 1) a consistent sound pattern or sign that approximates a conventional word; and 2) a form that is used to refer to a specific object, action, or attribute and only that word class. A word may be used either singly or in combination with a different word or an unintelligible string of sounds. The child needs to use a word only once spontaneously to be credited for it.

Table 5.3 Consonant sounds credited in the CSBS DP Behavior Sample

/m/	"mamamama" or "mama" or "moo"
/n/	"nununu" or "no no"
/b/ or /p/	"babababa" or "bibo" or "poo" or "bye bye"
/d/ or /t/	"dodododo" or "titi" or "daddy"
/g/ or /k/	"googoo" or "cookie" or "gone gone"
/w/	"woowoo" or " weewee" or "wagon"
/l/	"lalala" or "balloon" or "little"
/y/	"yayaya" or "yum yum" or "you"
/s/	"sasasa" or "sock" or "kiss"
/sh/	"shashasha" or "hush" or "shoe"

The child can also receive credit for a word that is imitated if the child uses that word a second time. Remember that only words used in communicative acts are to be credited. Scales 12 and 13 are a measure of the use of words and the number of different words that the child uses in communicative acts during the communication sample.

Scale 12 measures the child's use of at least one word in a sampling opportunity. The child's use of a word should be credited for each sampling opportunity. In contrast to Scale 13, for Scale 12, the variety of words should not influence the rating; that is, the child may use only one word, the same word many times, or many words, and be credited once for each sampling opportunity that a word is used.

Scale 13 is a measure of the variety of different words used by the child. Transcribe up to 16 different words used during the 6 sampling opportunities. Only transcribe new words that have not already been transcribed. This scale is not a measure of the child's entire vocabulary but an index of the variety of words used, up to 16 different words. For children who use a large number of different words, don't attempt to transcribe every word produced. Transcribe up to four different words per opportunity, if it is difficult to keep up with the child's productions.

Scales 14 and 15 are a measure of the use of word combinations and the number of different word combinations the child uses in communicative acts during the Behavior Sample. A *word combination* is defined as an utterance that contains at least two intelligible words; the words must be used either singly or in combination with a different word during the sample.

Scale 14 measures the child's use of at least one word combination in a communicative act. The child's use of a word combination should be credited for each sampling opportunity. In contrast to Scale 15, for Scale 14, the variety of word combinations should not influence the rating; that is, the child may use the same word combination many times and be credited once for each sampling opportunity that a word combination is used.

Scale 15 is a measure of the variety of different word combinations used by the child. Transcribe up to eight different word combinations used during the six sampling opportunities. Only transcribe new word combinations that have not already been transcribed. This scale is not a measure of the child's entire repertoire, but an index of the variety of word combinations used, up to eight different combinations.

SYMBOLIC BEHAVIOR SCALES

Scales 16–20 measure symbolic behaviors and are included as a global measure of the child's ability to use deliberate behavior and to plan ahead through mental representation and the use of symbols. There are five scales to measure different domains of symbolic representation. Scale 16 measures the understanding of words, and Scales 17–20 measure the use of objects.

Understanding

Scale 16 is a measure of language comprehension based on the language comprehension probes context. The evaluator should rate the child's comprehension of object names, person names, and body parts. The child's best comprehension response is rated. A countable response for language comprehension is touching, showing, or making a clear change in direction of eye gaze to correctly identify the objects, people, and body parts. The child can be credited a maximum of three object names, two person names, and three body parts.

Object Use

Scales 17–19 measure the quality of action schemes that the child uses during the symbolic play probes. An *action scheme* is defined as appropriate use of an object in the proper orientation toward an agent. An example of appropriate orientation and movement is holding the handle of the spoon. Correct top–bottom or front–back orientation is not necessary; that is, the concave side of the spoon does not need to be facing upward. The child may serve as the agent. Other possible agents include the two adults and the plush doll. An action scheme may be used singly or in sequences of two or more action schemes. On Scales 17–19, the child needs to use an action scheme only once spontaneously to be credited for it. The child can receive credit for using an action scheme if it was modeled by the adult and the child uses it with a different agent or different object or if it was in response to verbal directions of the adult without a model. The child can also receive credit for an action scheme that is an imitation using the same object and agent modeled by the adult but only if the child uses the action scheme a second time.

The following are the most common action schemes with the materials used in the symbolic play context.

1. Puts in
2. Puts on
3. Drinks with bottle
4. Drinks with cup
5. Hugs
6. Kisses
7. Feeds with utensil
8. Feeds with bowl
9. Stirs
10. Scoops
11. Pours

Note that we do distinguish between drinking with a bottle versus a cup but do not distinguish between feeding with the small spoon, big spoon, or spatula. The child can also be credited for variations on these action schemes (e.g., pats the plush doll instead of hugs; feeds with frying pan instead of bowl) and for one additional action scheme by writing it in space Number 12. For example, the action "blows on food to cool it off" is one we have seen a few children use but not enough to include in the list of 11 common actions. This action would be written in Number 12.

Scale 17 is a measure of the inventory of different action schemes that the child uses during the symbolic play context. The variety of different action schemes that the child uses toward self or other should be noted up to a total of 12 different actions. Make a check in the appropriate box next to the action displayed. A child is credited for each different action scheme used, regardless of the agent. For example, if the child feeds self and feeds the doll with the spoon, credit the child once for the action scheme of feeds with utensil for Scale 17. Similar actions with different objects are sometimes credited as different action schemes. For example, if the child drinks with the bottle and drinks with the cup, the child is credited for two different action schemes.

Scales 18 and 19 are a measure of the complexity of the child's use of agents and actions with objects during the symbolic play context. Two aspects of the complexity of the child's use of action schemes are measured: in Scale 18, the use of action schemes toward self versus other agents; and in Scale 19, the use of different action schemes used singly versus in sequence. For Scale 18, possible agents include the child, the two adults, and the plush doll. For each action scheme that the child uses toward an agent other than him- or herself, credit the child by indicating the number in Scale 17 corresponding with the action scheme (e.g., 7 for feeds with utensil) and the initials of the agent. For example, if the child feeds the plush doll with a spoon, credit the child by recording "7 PD" in the first space (*PD* refers to plush doll). The child can be credited once for each different action scheme used with each different agent. For example, if the child offers the bottle to the plush doll and his or her mother, then credit the child with two actions toward other by recording "3 PD" in the first space and "3 M" (*M* stands for mom) in the second space.

An action scheme may be used singly or in sequences of two or more action schemes. A multiple-action scheme is the combination of two or more different single-action schemes used successively, whether directed toward self or other. Note that using the same single-action scheme with more than one agent is not considered a multiple-action scheme. In other words, *a multiple-action scheme must involve at least two different action schemes combined in sequence.* However, the sequence need not be logical or related in theme; that is, the order in which the two (or more) action schemes are used does not have to be the order in which a person would perform the same actions in natural feeding or grooming routines. In fact, use of logical sequence in multiple-action schemes does not usually appear until after age 24 months.

For each multiple-action scheme that the child uses, credit the child by indicating the sequences of numbers corresponding with the multiple-action scheme. The following are two examples of multiple-action schemes.

- Stir in bowl, feed doll with spoon (credit child by recording 9+7)
- Stir in bowl, pour into cup, and give doll drink with cup (credit child by recording 9+11+4)

For Scales 18 and 19, a child can be credited for use of up to six different action schemes toward other and six different sequences of action schemes. If the child uses the same action scheme or sequence of action schemes more than once, the child should only be credited once.

Scale 20 is a measure of the child's ability to use one object in combination with another object or group of objects to construct a product (e.g., tower). This aspect of play should be influenced the least by the child's social and communicative abilities and thus should provide a relatively pure measure of nonverbal mental representation ability. The blocks used during the constructive play context provide the child with the opportunity to use objects that do not require an ordinal relation. The highest number of blocks stacked should be recorded. Combinatorial actions with the blocks may include stacking or lining up. Taking blocks off a stack, mouthing, or banging objects together does not count as a combinatorial action. The child is credited with 1 point for trying to stack but failing because the block falls off. The child is credited with 2–5 points for stacking 2–5 blocks, respectively.

RATING BEHAVIORS ON THE BEHAVIOR SAMPLE: SCORING WORKSHEET

The CSBS DP Behavior Sample: Scoring Worksheet is to be completed while collecting the CSBS DP Behavior Sample or while watching a videotape of the Behavior Sample with minimal stopping of the tape. Begin by rating behaviors observed during the first sampling opportunity.

For the first two scales, record the presence of gaze shifts and shared positive affect with a √ or +. Skip to Scale 4, and record rate of communicating by circling either 0, 1, 2, or 3+ to indicate that the child displayed no acts, one act, two acts, or three or more acts, respectively. It may help to put a small check above the numbers 1, 2, and 3 as the child displays communicative acts during the sampling opportunity and then circle the highest number of communicative acts displayed at the end of the sampling opportunity.

For Scales 5–7, record the presence of behavior regulation, social interaction, and joint attention with a √ or +. The child may display more than one instance of each function but only one check per function is to be recorded per samplingopportunity.

For conventional gestures (Scale 8), check all of the gestures that the child used during this sampling opportunity and compare them from the list of conventional gestures. For distal gestures (Scale 9), record the presence with a √ or +.

Proceed to Scales 10 and 11. For syllables with consonants, record the presence with a √ or +. For inventory of consonants, check all the different consonants that the child used during this sampling opportunity from the list of consonants.

For Scales 12 and 14, record the presence of a word or word combination in a communicative act during this sampling opportunity with a √ or +. In addition, transcribe orthographically or phonetically up to 16 different words for Scale 13 and eight different word combinations for Scale 15. For children who produce a large number of words and word combinations during the sample, transcribe about four different words and two different word combinations per opportunity.

For the second sampling opportunity, begin at the top of column 2 and record the presence of each communication scale parameter for each communicative opportunity until the end of Sampling Opportunity 6 as described previously. Record the gaze/point following probes immediately after administering them at the end of Sampling Opportunities 2 and 5.

The next step is to complete the Symbolic Behavior Scales. Record language comprehension, Scale 16, beginning with object names as the toys from the symbolic play probes are being put away. Record the correct identification of object names, person names, and body parts by putting a check or plus and writing the name in the spaces provided on the worksheet. Leave the space blank or put a minus next to the name if the child failed to demonstrate comprehension. We find that writing the name is important for keeping track of trials and handling repeated trials, which may be presented out of order.

Rate symbolic play probes by first checking the inventory of different action schemes demonstrated during this context for single-action schemes toward self, single-action schemes toward other, or multiple-action schemes. For Scale 17, check the number of different action schemes. If the child displays an action scheme that is not listed, write that action in the empty space provided. For Scale 18, indicate whether the child directed the action scheme toward another agent (either the plush doll, caregiver, or evaluator) by recording the action number (from Scale 17) and the initials of the agent for up to six different action schemes. For Scale 19, indicate whether the child combined different action schemes by recording the sequence of action numbers (from Scale 17) for up to six different sequences of action schemes.

For Scale 20, record the greatest number of blocks stacked by circling 0, 1, 2, 3, 4, or 5 to indicate how many blocks the child stacked successfully. Remember to record the presence of each parameter of the Communicative Scales as well as each parameter of the Symbolic Behaviors Scales for Sampling Opportunity 6 from the beginning of the symbolic play until the end of the blocks.

COMPLETING THE CSBS DP BEHAVIOR SAMPLE: SCORING SUMMARY

The CSBS DP Behavior Sample consists of 20 scales within each of the seven clusters. The scoring process consists of five steps. The first step is to sum the points for each scale and to compute the weighted raw scores for each cluster. The second step is to sum the seven cluster weighted raw scores to obtain the weighted raw scores for each of the three composite scores. The third step is to sum the three composite weighted raw scores to obtain the total weighted raw score. The fourth step is to convert the weighted raw scores to normed scores. The fifth step is to interpret and report the normed scores.

Step 1: Sum the points for each item and obtain the weighted raw scores for each of the seven clusters.

Give credit of 1 point for all responses that are present for each sampling opportunity and no points for absences. For Scale 4, rate of communicating, give credit of 0, 1, 2, or 3 points for all rates of *0*, *1*, *2*, or *3+*, respectively. Give credit of 1 point for each item checked from the checklist format for inventory of conventional gestures, consonants, and action schemes and credit of 1 point for each word and word combination transcribed. The point values and total possible points are listed in Table 5.4.

The number of points earned should be totaled to yield weighted raw scores for each of the seven clusters. The scales should be tallied on CSBS DP Behavior Sample: Scoring Worksheet. Scales 3, 4, 8, 11, 13, and 16 are weighted by dividing or multiplying by a factor of 2 or 3, and the weighting factor is indicated on the worksheet and in Table 5.4. Weighting certain scales was done in order to make the point value

Table 5.4. Point values of each scale, weighting, and total possible weighted points for each cluster on the Behavior Sample

Cluster	Possible points	Weighting	Weighted points
Emotion and Eye Gaze			
Scale 1	6		6
Scale 2	6		6
Scale 3	2	Multiply by 3	6
Total			**18**
Communication			
Scale 4	18	Divide by 3	6
Scale 5	6		6
Scale 6	6		6
Scale 7	6		6
Total			**24**
Gestures			
Scale 8	8	Multiply by 2	16
Scale 9	6		6
Total			**22**
Sounds			
Scale 10	6		6
Scale 11	10	Multiply by 2	20
Total			**26**
Words			
Scale 12	6		6
Scale 13	16	Divide by 2	8
Scale 14	6		6
Scale 15	8		8
Total			**28**
Understanding			
Scale 16			
Object names	3	Multiply by 3	9
Person names	2	Multiply by 3	6
Body Parts	3	Multiply by 3	9
Total			**24**
Object use			
Scale 17	12		12
Scale 18	6		6
Scale 19	6		6
Scale 20	5		5
Total			**29**

across scales and clusters comparable. The value of the scales with weighting should be tallied more carefully, with particular attention to the weighting factor. Then, the weighted raw scores should be summed for each cluster.

Step 2: Sum the seven cluster weighted raw scores to obtain the weighted raw scores for each of the three composites.

The seven clusters are organized into three composites—Social, Speech, and Symbolic. The second step is to sum the seven cluster weighted raw scores to obtain the three composite weighted raw scores. The seven cluster weighted raw scores tallied on the CSBS DP Behavior Sample: Scoring Worksheet should be transferred to the column labeled *Weighted Raw Score* on the CSBS DP Behavior Sample: Scoring Summary. These seven cluster weighted raw scores should be summed to yield the weighted raw scores for the three composites. That is, the weighted raw score for the Social Composite is the sum of the Emotion and Eye Gaze, Communication, and Gestures Clusters. The weighted raw score for the Speech Composite is the sum of the Sounds and Words Clusters. The weighted raw score for the Symbolic Composite is the sum of the Understanding and Object Use Clusters. The composite weighted raw scores should be tallied in the column labeled *Weighted Raw Score* under the cluster weighted raw scores on the CSBS DP Behavior Sample: Scoring Summary. The total possible points for the weighted raw scores of the three composites are listed in Table 5.5.

Step 3: Sum the three composite weighted raw scores to obtain the total weighted raw score.

The third step is to sum the three composite weighted raw scores on the Behavior Sample: Scoring Summary to obtain the total weighted raw score. The total weighted raw score should be tallied at the bottom of the column labeled *Weighted Raw Score* on the Behavior Sample: Scoring Summary, just below the composite weighted raw scores. The total possible points for the total weighted raw score are listed in Table 5.5.

Step 4: Convert the cluster, composite, and total weighted raw scores to normed scores.

The fourth step is to convert the cluster, composite, and total weighted raw scores to normed scores. Normed scores are provided in the norms tables for the CSBS DP Behavior Sample in Appendix C and are based on chronological age to reflect the performance of children in the standardization sample from 12 to 24 months with the following intervals: 12–14 months, 15–17 months, 18–20 months, and 21–24 months.

Table 5.5. Total possible points for each cluster, composite, and total on the Behavior Sample

Composite	Possible points
Social Composite	
Emotion and Eye Gaze	18
Communication	24
Gestures	22
Total	**64**
Speech Composite	
Sounds	26
Words	28
Total	**54**
Symbolic Composite	
Understanding	24
Object Use	29
Total	**53**
Social Composite	64
Speech Composite	54
Symbolic Composite	53
Total	**171**

Use the following steps to compute the child's chronological age:

1. Enter the child's name, date filled out, and date of birth on the CSBS DP Behavior Sample: Scoring Worksheet. If the child is more than 4 weeks premature, make sure to enter the child's corrected date of birth and indicate this by writing *corrected* in parentheses after the date of birth and chronological age.
2. If the child is more than 4 weeks premature, compute the child's chronological age on the Behavior Sample: Scoring Worksheet by subtracting the child's date of birth (month, day, and year) from the date of completion (month, day, and year).
3. Subtract days first, then months, then years. Table 5.6 shows a simple subtraction in which no borrowing is required.
4. If the day of the month on which the child was born is larger than the day of the month of testing, borrow 30 days; that is, add 30 days to the day of testing and subtract 1 month from the month of testing. If necessary, also borrow 1 month of testing by adding 12 months to the actual month of testing and subtracting 1 year from the testing year. Table 5.7 shows a subtraction in which borrowing is required for a child whose date of completion was November 5, 2000.
5. The child's chronological age should be reported in months, and the month should not be rounded up. For example, a child is 12 months old from 12 months and 0 days until that child turns 13 months and 0 days. To calculate age in months, first multiply the number of years by 12, and then add the number of extra months. The chronological age for the child in Table 5.6 is 16 months (i.e., multiply 1 for the number of years by 12 and add 4 extra months to get 16) and would not be rounded to 17 months, even though the child is more than 16 $^1/_2$ months old. The chronological age for the child in Table 5.7 is 21 months.

Standard scores and percentile ranks are the normed scores provided in the norms tables for the clusters, composites, and total for the CSBS DP Behavior Sample in Appendix C. The standard scores for the seven clusters and three composites are based on a mean of 10 and a standard deviation of 3. The standard scores for the total are based on a mean of 100 and a standard deviation of 15. Because standard scores reflect equal units of measurement, they may be added, subtracted, or averaged. A percentile rank reflects the percentage of children in the sample scoring at or below a given raw score. Percentile ranks, unlike standard scores, should not be added, subtracted, or averaged. Standard scores, rather than percentile ranks, should be used to reflect average performance, whether it is the average of several scores for an individual child or the average of scores obtained from a group of children. The relationship between the standard scores and percentile ranks is shown in Table 5.8.

Table 5.6. Calculating chronological age without needing to borrow

	Month	Day	Year
Date of completion	10	25	2000
Date of birth	6	4	1999
Chronological age	**4**	**21**	**1**
CSBS DP age	**16**		

Table 5.7. Calculating chronological age with borrowing

	Month	Day	Year
Date of completion	~~11~~ 10	~~5~~ 35	2000
Date of birth	1	28	1999
Chronological age	**9**	**7**	**1**
CSBS DP age	**9**		

Table 5.8. Standard deviations (SD), standard scores (SS), and percentile ranks (%ile) for the clusters, composites, and total scores

SD	Cluster and composite SS	Total SS	%ile
	17	135	99
+2 SD	16	130	98
	15	125	95
	14	120	91
+1 SD	13	115	84
	12	110	75
	11	105	63
Mean	10	100	50
	9	95	37
	8	90	25
-1 SD	7	85	16
	6	80	9
	5	75	5
-2 SD	4	70	2
	3	65	1

Once the child's chronological age is known, use the following steps to look up the standard scores and percentile ranks for the clusters, composites, and total weighted raw scores. Use the norms tables for the CSBS DP Behavior Sample in Appendix C. On the table for the Emotion and Eye Gaze Cluster, find the column with the child's chronological age in months. Read down the column until you find the child's Emotion and Eye Gaze Cluster weighted raw score, and look to the left to find the corresponding standard score (SS) and percentile rank (%ile). Enter these scores in the appropriate columns on the Behavior Sample: Scoring Summary. (*Note:* If the Behavior Sample is being used to monitor change for children who are older than 24 months of age, use the oldest normative group, which is 21–24 months for comparison purposes but document this when reporting results.) Repeat this for the other six clusters, the three composites, and the total.

Step 5: Interpret and report the normed scores.

The fifth and last step is to interpret and report the normed scores. Once the child's standard scores and percentile ranks are entered, use the following steps to determine if the normed scores are of concern and decide what to recommend.

Determine if the normed scores are of concern and enter *Yes* in the column labeled *concern*. There are 11 scores that may fall in a range of concern or no concern—the seven clusters, the three composites, and the total. We have set the criterion level for concern for the composite and total scores based on performance of at least 1.25 standard deviations below the mean as follows:

- Standard scores at or below 6 for the clusters and composites
- Standard scores at or below 81 for the total score
- Percentile ranks at or below the 10th for the composites and total scores

Compare the normed scores on the CSBS DP Behavior Sample with those obtained from the CSBS DP Caregiver Questionnaire.

The CSBS DP Behavior Sample can be used to monitor development every 3 months between 12 and 24 months. Because it is based on a face-to-face evaluation, it is possible to underestimate the child's abilities because the child may be apprehensive, anxious, shy, or uncooperative. Therefore, this tool should be used along with information provided by the parent about what the child can do. Although eligibility criteria for receiving services vary from state to state, it is recommended that children who have scores in the concern range on at least three clusters, any composite, or the total score be considered at-risk for a developmental delay or disability. If a consistent pattern is also documented on the CSBS DP Caregiver Questionnaire, that child should be referred for a diagnostic evaluation and/or further assessment to plan support or intervention services. If there is a discrepancy between the pattern of scores on the Behavior Sample and the Caregiver Questionnaire, reasons for this discrepancy should be considered (i.e., Is the parent over- or under-estimating the child's performance, or is the child performing below potential on the behavior sample?).

The CSBS DP Behavior Sample should only be used along with the CSBS DP Caregiver Questionnaire to decide whether a child is developmentally delayed. Caution should be taken not to alarm parents. We find that many parents already have concerns about their children, especially if their children are about 18 months old and are behind in language development. The early intervention literature emphasizes the notion of multiple risk factors; therefore, a child's scores on this Behavior Sample need to be considered in relation to other known biological or environmental risk factors. Clinical judgment should be used in making decisions about the need for further evaluation with these cutoffs as guidelines. Remember that the Behavior Sample is not meant for a diagnostic evaluation and should not be used for a differential diagnosis.

6 SAMPLING AND SCORING TUTORIAL FOR THE CSBS DP BEHAVIOR SAMPLE

The sampling and scoring procedures for the CSBS DP Behavior Sample may seem daunting for novice evaluators. Therefore, this chapter is designed to serve as a self-tutorial for sampling and scoring procedures. This chapter accompanies the two tutorial videotapes included in the CSBS DP kit, which feature six typically developing children. The reader should first read the notes in this chapter about each Behavior Sample session and then view the sample two times, the first time to reflect on the sampling procedures and the second time to try to score the sample. Reflections on our sampling procedures and explanations about our scoring decisions are provided for each sample.

OVERVIEW OF THE TUTORIAL CHAPTER

The purpose of this tutorial chapter is to provide you with the opportunity to visualize the flow of the sampling procedures and to calibrate your CSBS DP scoring. The tutorial consists of this chapter and the two CSBS DP videotapes. Each videotape contains three samples of typically developing children, who range in age from 12 to 21 months. The completed Behavior Sample: Scoring Worksheets for these six children and detailed comments explaining our scoring decisions are included in this chapter. This chapter and the accompanying videotapes were designed to take you step-by-step through the sampling and scoring procedures and decisions. You will have an opportunity to score each of the six samples. By viewing and scoring the samples on the videotape, you will be able to compare your approach to sampling and scoring with ours and understand our decision-making process for administering and scoring the CSBS DP.

Calibrating your scoring is a gradual process of adjusting and refining your decision-making. It may be helpful to review the *CSBS Manual, Normed Edition* (Wetherby & Prizant, 1993), the CSBS Scoring Videotape (Wetherby, Prizant, & Barnes, 1993), and the CSBS Scoring Tutorial Videotape (Wetherby, Prizant, & Kublin, 1995). These resources provide a basic understanding of the parameters measured with the CSBS.

Scoring the CSBS DP Behavior Sample entails interpreting the child's behavior in relation to definitions presented in the manual. Unlike other formal assessment instruments, there may not be only one correct answer when scoring a particular communicative act or behavior. It is important that you understand our scoring decisions because the scoring decisions for the normed sample were based on this decision-making process.

We recognize the amount of time required to learn to score CSBS DP Behavior Sample. It is our hope that the effort you put into learning to score the Behavior

Sample will enhance your clinical skills. Based on feedback from clinicians and advanced students, we are confident that learning to score the Behavior Sample will help you improve your clinical skills in the following ways:

1. To develop your ability to analyze interactions of young children by providing a framework for observation
2. To expand the knowledge base that you can draw on about early interaction skills
3. To enhance your ability to make judgments regarding a child's communicative and symbolic profile while interacting with that child

HOW TO USE THIS TUTORIAL

We recommend that you watch the six samples in the order presented on the videotape. You should begin this tutorial by viewing the first sample on the CSBS DP tutorial videotape. Camille (Mimi), 21 months of age, is the first child shown on the tape. First, view the sample to become familiar with the sampling procedures. Next, review the videotape to consider the decision-making process for completing the CSBS DP Behavior Sample: Scoring Worksheet available in the forms packet. You will need a blank record form for each sample.

For each child's sample, begin by viewing the first sampling opportunity (i.e., the wind-up toy and the toys in a bag), and then pause the videotape. Score Scales 1–15 on the worksheet. Then, check your scoring with the completed record forms and scoring explanations provided in this chapter. For any parameters you disagreed with, review that segment of the videotape and refer to the completed record forms and the scoring explanations.

Next, view the second sampling opportunity and pause the videotape. Score Scales 1–15, and check your scoring with the completed record forms in this chapter. You should continue scoring each sample, opportunity by opportunity, until you reach Opportunity 6: Play. For the last sample opportunity in the group, score Scales 1–20. It is *not* expected that you will agree on all scores because scoring decisions are based on the scorer's interpretations of each child's behavior. You are striving to achieve agreement on at least 8 of 10 scoring decisions or at a level of 80% reported in the manual for every parameter.

Each child's completed CSBS DP Behavior Sample: Scoring Worksheet is complemented with comments, including points to notice about the sampling procedures and the scoring decisions. We do not include comments about the scoring decisions made for every communicative act. Instead, we highlight important things to notice and learn from each child. We include many examples of communicative acts. For each of these acts, the number of the sampling opportunity is given to assist the viewer in identifying the particular act (e.g., #1 indicating wind-up toy, #3 indicating bubbles, #6 indicating play). Keep in mind that the CSBS DP encourages clinicians to make scoring decisions at the end of each communicative opportunity rather than for each communicative act. You need to learn to make quick decisions about whether the child displayed an example of each of the particular parameters. In learning the parameters, you will need to reflect on particular communicative acts. In scoring samples, however, you need to learn to make more comprehensive judgments. Give credit to the child only when the behaviors are clear examples of the parameters measured.

CAMILLE (MIMI): 21 MONTHS

Comments on Sampling Procedures

Camille (Mimi) used primarily verbal communication that was augmented with gaze shifts, shared affect, and gestures. In general, communicating for joint attention may be more difficult to sample and identify in scoring than behavior regulation or social interaction. Camille's sample, however, offers many examples of communicating for joint attention. Notice that the clinician and mother used a facilitative style of interacting with her by waiting, allowing her to initiate, and following her lead, usually by imitating or expanding on what she said. This facilitative style is optimal in collecting a communication sample, particularly to ensure that a child uses joint attention, and should be emulated. Notice how playful the interaction was with a lot of opportunities to share positive affect. The clinician made very smooth transitions from opportunity to opportunity by saying "Bye-bye," removing the object, and quickly bringing out the next object.

Comments on Scoring Decisions

Figure 6.1 shows a completed CSBS DP Behavior Sample: Scoring Worksheet for Camille. Camille displayed frequent gaze shifts and shared positive affect during this sample and was credited for each of these for every opportunity. She displayed many more than three communicative acts during each opportunity. She communicated numerous times for behavior regulation and joint attention but only once for social interaction. The following are some good examples of communicative acts used by Camille.

Behavior Regulation

#1: She said, "Table," when she wanted the clinician to put the wind-up duck on the table.

#1: Camille gave the duck to her mom to request winding it up.

#3: She reached toward the clinician and said, "Doggie," to request the dog figure that had been put away.

Social Interaction

#4: She raised her arms to be picked up or hugged while leaning toward her mother and said, "Up," to request comfort.

Joint Attention

#1: Camille said, "Running," to comment on the duck.

#1: She said, "Little Bird," while pointing to draw attention to the small figure of Big Bird holding Little Bird (Big Bird/Little Bird figure).

CSBS DP

CSBS DP Behavior Sample: Scoring Worksheet

Child's name: Camille

Date completed: 7-14-01

Date of birth: 10-4-99

Chronological age[1]: 21 months

[1] If child is 4 or more weeks premature, use corrected age. Calculate chronological age by subtracting Date of birth from Date the Behavior Sample was completed.

Sampling Opportunity:	1	2	3	4	5	6
	Wind-up toy	*Balloon*	*Bubbles*	*Jar*	*Books*	*Play*

COMMUNICATION SCALES (Score during Opportunities 1 to 6)

Emotion and Eye Gaze

	1	2	3	4	5	6
1. Gaze shifts	☒	☒	☒	☒	☒	☒
2. Shared positive affect	☒	☒	☒	☒	☒	☐
3. Gaze/point following		☒			☒	

Weighted Raw Score: Scale 1 [6] + Scale 2 [5] + Scale 3 2 × 3 [6] = **17**

Communication

	1	2	3	4	5	6
4. Rate of communicating	✓✓ 0 1 2 (3+)	✓✓ 0 1 2 (3+)	✓✓ 0 1 2 (3+)	✓✓ 0 1 2 (3+)	✓✓ 0 1 2 (3+)	✓✓ 0 1 2 (3+)
5. Behavior regulation	☒	☒	☒	☒	☒	☒
6. Social interaction	☐	☐	☐	☒	☒	☐
7. Joint attention	☒	☒	☒	☒	☒	☒

Weighted Raw Score: Scale 4 18 ÷ 3 [6] + Scale 5 [6] + Scale 6 [2] + Scale 7 [6] = **20**

Gestures

8. Inventory of conventional gestures
check all that child uses:

☒ gives	☒ shows	☒ pushes/pulls away	☒ reaches
☒ points	☐ waves	☒ nods head	☒ shakes head

	1	2	3	4	5	6
9. Distal gestures	☒	☐	☒	☒	☒	☐

Weighted Raw Score: Scale 8 7 × 2 [14] + Scale 9 [4] = **18**

Sounds

	1	2	3	4	5	6
10. Syllables with consonants	☒	☒	☒	☒	☒	☒

11. Inventory of consonants
check all that child uses:

☒ /m/	☒ /n/	☒ /blp/	☒ /dlt/	☒ /glk/
☒ /w/	☐ /t/	☐ /y/	☒ /s/	☒ /sh/

Weighted Raw Score: Scale 10 [6] + Scale 11 8 × 2 [16] = **22**

Words

	1	2	3	4	5	6
12. Words	☒	☒	☒	☒	☒	☒

13. Inventory of words
write examples of words used:

table 1	running 2	Mimi 3	wind it 4
toes 5	other way 6	walking 7	birdie 8
again 9	doggie 10	bubble 11	open 12
no 13	Dot Dot's 14	Hannah's 15	bag 16

	1	2	3	4	5	6
14. Word combinations	☒	☒	☒	☒	☒	☒

15. Inventory of word combinations
write examples of words combined:

Little Bird 1	no doggie 2
see it 3	no hand 4
mine's home 5	Mickey Mouse eating 6
not that 7	stir it 8

Weighted Raw Score: Scale 12 [6] + Scale 13 16 ÷ 2 [8] + Scale 14 [6] + Scale 15 [8] = **28**

Figure 6.1. Completed CSBS DP Behavior Sample: Scoring Worksheet for Camille.

SYMBOLIC BEHAVIOR SCALES (Score only during Opportunity 6 Play)

Understanding

16. Language comprehension

	1	2	3	4
object names:	spoon X	bottle X	cup X	
person names:	Mom X	Mimi X		
body parts:	eyes X	nose X	hair X	ears X

(maximum of 3 raw score) (maximum of 2 raw score) (maximum of 3 raw score)

Weighted Raw Score: *Object names* 3 × 3 [9] + *Person names* 2 × 3 [6] + *Body parts* 3 × 3 [9] = [24]

Object Use

17. Inventory of action schemes

check all that child uses:

❑ puts in [1]	☒ puts on [2]	☒ drinks with bottle [3]	☒ drinks with cup [4]	❑ hugs [5]	❑ kisses [6]
☒ feeds with utensil [7]	❑ feeds with bowl [8]	☒ stirs [9]	☒ scoops [10]	☒ pours [11]	other action: ☒ stands up [12]

18. Action schemes toward other

write action numbers & agent's initials:

12 BB	3 BB	7 BB			

19. Sequences action schemes

write action numbers:

9 + 7	11 + 2	10 + 7	11 + 2	11 + 9	11 + 4

20. Stacks tower of blocks

circle highest number:

refuses, mouths, or bangs	tries but fails to stack	stacks	stacks	stacks	stacks
0	1	2	3	4	(5)

Weighted Raw Score: Scale 17 [8] + Scale 18 [3] + Scale 19 [6] + Scale 20 [5] = [22]

CSBS DP™ Behavior Sample: Scoring Summary

		Weighted raw score	Standard score	Percentile rank	Concern
Cluster scores					
Social	Emotion and Eye Gaze	17	14	91	
	Communication	20	12	75	
	Gestures	18	13	84	
Speech	Sounds	22	12	75	
	Words	28	17	99	
Symbolic	Understanding	24	17	99	
	Object Use	22	14	91	
Composite scores					
	Social	55	14	91	
	Speech	50	14	91	
	Symbolic	46	15	95	
TOTAL		151	135	99	

#3: After pulling the foot-shaped teether out of the bag, she showed it to her mom and said, "See it?"

#6: After putting the lid on the bowl, she said, "Hot hot." (Notice that the first time Camille said, "Hot hot," it was not counted as a communicative act because it was not directed. Then, her mom said, "Hot dogs." Camille clarified what she was saying by repeating "hot hot" while looking at her mom. This second production of "hot hot" was a nice example of joint attention.)

Camille used many conventional gestures throughout the sample but a few were subtle and could be easily missed. For example, she used a pull away gesture when she gave the duck to her mom and then pulled the duck away while saying, "Mimi," indicating she wanted it back. She used only a few distal gestures. One example of a distal gesture was when she depicted the duck walking by shaking her hands (she did this first while holding the duck, which would not be considered distal). Another example was when she reached toward the clinician while saying, "Doggie," to request the dog figure that was out of reach. This action was followed by a contact point on the table to indicate where the clinician should put the dog.

Camille used many sounds during the sample, most within words. She used the nasals and plosives frequently. She used the /w/ in *wind it*, the /sh/ as the final consonant in *toes*, and the /s/ as the possessive ending in *Dot Dot's* and *Hannah's*. Camille used primarily single words to communicate throughout the sample. She used a few word combinations, but these were only counted if the words were also used singly or in other combinations. For example, *Little Bird* was counted as a word combination because she used *Birdie* separately. *Wind it*, *other way*, and *blow 'em* were not counted as word combinations because she had not used those individual words separately or in other combinations. *No doggie* was counted as a word combination because she had used *doggie* and *no* singly.

Camille displayed excellent symbolic behaviors. She demonstrated language comprehension for all items tested. She demonstrated a large variety of action schemes, including making the Big Bird doll stand up. She used several actions toward the Big Bird doll and put more than six sequences of actions together. She was able to stack all five blocks.

ABBY: 20 MONTHS

Comments on Sampling Procedures

Abby used primarily verbal communication but initially was not very cooperative. This behavior is common for young children, particularly between ages 15 and 20 months, when they are given instructions requiring compliance (e.g., "Sit here"). The clinician was able to work through this situation easily by giving Abby choices and following her lead. Notice that the pace of the sample allowed Abby to contemplate each opportunity as it was presented, and the clinician responded to Abby's communication by imitating or expanding on what she said. Abby began to leave the table several times, and the clinician was able to get her to return by enticing her with the materials for the next opportunity and telling her that she needed to sit down in order to play with the materials.

Comments on Scoring Decisions

Figure 6.2 shows a completed CSBS DP Behavior Sample: Scoring Worksheet for Abby. Like Camille, Abby displayed frequent gaze shifts and shared positive affect and communication during this sample. She displayed many more than three communicative acts during each opportunity. In addition, she communicated numerous times for behavior regulation and joint attention but only once for social interaction. Here are some good examples of communicative acts used by Abby:

Behavior Regulation

#2: Abby said, "Mommy," while giving the balloon to her mom to request her to blow it up.

#2: She used an open-hand reach toward the balloon when it was first brought out to request it. (This is also credited for distal gesture.)

#2: She said, "Mine," and pulled the duck away in response to the clinician asking, "Are you all done with Mr. Duck?"

#3: Abby said, "Bubble," to request that the clinician open the jar of bubbles.

#3: She said, "Blow bubba," while pointing to the wand in response to her mom saying, "What should I do?" (This was credited for word combination.)

Social Interaction

#4: Abby said, "Thank you," after getting Cheerios as an acknowledgment. (The first two times she said, "Thank you," were not directed, but the third was with eye gaze.) This exchange was considered social interaction because she was directing attention to herself rather than to the object.

Joint Attention

#2: She imitated *all gone* while putting the balloon away. (This was not counted as a word because it was imitated.)

#2: She said, "A duck," after pulling the Koosh duck out of the bag. (This was counted as a word but not a word combination because she had not used either word separately or in another combination.)

#5: Abby said, "Bug," while pointing to a picture of a bug in the book.

During the language comprehension probe, the clinician presented four trials of object names, as specified in the sampling procedures. Abby responded correctly to the first trial (spoon), missed the second (cup) and third (bowl) trials, and got the fourth trial (bottle) correct. She thus achieved credit of 2 for object names. She received the maximum credit of 2 and 3, respectively, for person names and body parts.

During symbolic play, she scooped with the spoon and fed the Big Bird doll. Then, she stirred with the spoon and fed the Big Bird doll. The difference between her scoop and stir was that her scoop had only a single swiping motion and her stir

CSBS DP

CSBS DP Behavior Sample: Scoring Worksheet

Child's name: *Abby*

Date completed: *5-19-01*

Date of birth: *9-16-99*

Chronological age[1]: *20 months*

[1] If child is 4 or more weeks premature, use corrected age. Calculate chronological age by subtracting Date of birth from Date the Behavior Sample was completed.

	1	2	3	4	5	6
Sampling Opportunity:	Wind-up toy	Balloon	Bubbles	Jar	Books	Play

COMMUNICATION SCALES (Score during Opportunities 1 to 6)

Emotion and Eye Gaze

	1	2	3	4	5	6
1. Gaze shifts	☒	☒	☒	☒	☒	☒
2. Shared positive affect	☒	☒	☒	☐	☒	☒
3. Gaze/point following		☒			☒	

Weighted Raw Score: Scale 1 [6] + Scale 2 [5] + Scale 3 _2_ × 3 [6] = **17**

Communication

	1	2	3	4	5	6
4. Rate of communicating	✓✓ 0 1 2 (3+)	✓✓ 0 1 2 (3+)	✓✓ 0 1 2 (3+)	✓✓ 0 1 2 (3+)	✓✓ 0 1 2 (3+)	✓✓ 0 1 2 (3+)
5. Behavior regulation	☒	☒	☒	☒	☒	☒
6. Social interaction	☐	☐	☐	☒	☐	☐
7. Joint attention	☒	☒	☒	☐	☒	☒

Weighted Raw Score: Scale 4 _18_ ÷ 3 [6] + Scale 5 [6] + Scale 6 [1] + Scale 7 [5] = **18**

Gestures

8. Inventory of conventional gestures
check all that child uses:

☒ gives	☒ shows	☒ pushes/pulls away	☒ reaches
☒ points	☒ waves	☒ nods head	☒ shakes head

	1	2	3	4	5	6
9. Distal gestures	☐	☒	☒	☒	☒	☒

Weighted Raw Score: Scale 8 _7_ × 2 [14] + Scale 9 [5] = **19**

Sounds

	1	2	3	4	5	6
10. Syllables with consonants	☒	☒	☒	☒	☒	☒

11. Inventory of consonants
check all that child uses:

☒ /m/	☒ /n/	☒ /b|p/	☒ /d|t/	☐ /g|k/
☒ /w/	☒ /t/	☐ /y/	☐ /s/	☐ /sh/

Weighted Raw Score: Scale 10 [6] + Scale 11 _6_ × 2 [12] = **18**

Words

	1	2	3	4	5	6
12. Words	☒	☒	☒	☒	☒	☒

13. Inventory of words
write examples of words used:

uh oh 1	*ball* 2	*mine* 3	*Mommy* 4
no 5	*a duck* 6	*bubble* 7	*thank you* 8
dog 9	*that yellow* 10	*down* 11	*bug* 12
more 13	*hat* 14	*whoo* 15	16

	1	2	3	4	5	6
14. Word combinations	☐	☐	☒	☐	☐	☐

15. Inventory of word combinations
write examples of words combined:

blow bubble 1	2
3	4
5	6
7	8

Weighted Raw Score: Scale 12 [6] + Scale 13 _15_ ÷ 2 [8] + Scale 14 [1] + Scale 15 [1] = **16**

Figure 6.2. Completed CSBS DP Behavior Sample: Scoring Worksheet for Abby.

SYMBOLIC BEHAVIOR SCALES (Score only during Opportunity 6 Play)

Understanding

16. Language comprehension

object names:	X spoon [1]	cup [2]	bowl [3]	X bottle [4]
person names:	X Mom [1]	X Mickey [2]	[3]	
body parts:	X eyes [1]	X nose [2]	X hair [3]	[4]

(maximum of 3 raw score) (maximum of 2 raw score) (maximum of 3 raw score)

Weighted Raw Score: *Object names* 2 × 3 [6] + *Person Names* 2 × 3 [6] + *Body Parts* 3 × 3 [9] = [21]

Object Use

17. Inventory of action schemes
check all that child uses:

☒ puts in [1]	❑ puts on [2]	☒ drinks with bottle [3]	❑ drinks with cup [4]	❑ hugs [5]	❑ kisses [6]
☒ feeds with utensil [7]	❑ feeds with bowl [8]	☒ stirs [9]	☒ scoops [10]	☒ pours [11]	other action: ❑ [12]

18. Action schemes toward other
write action numbers & agent's initials:

7 BB	3 BB	3 Mom	3 CI		

19. Sequences action schemes
write action numbers:

10 + 7	9 + 7				

20. Stacks tower of blocks
circle highest number:

refuses, mouths, or bangs	tries but fails to stack	stacks	stacks	stacks	stacks
0	1	2	3	4	(5)

Weighted Raw Score: Scale 17 [6] + Scale 18 [4] + Scale 19 [2] + Scale 20 [5] = [17]

CSBS DP

CSBS DP Behavior Sample: Scoring Summary

		Weighted raw score	Standard score	Percentile rank	Concern
Cluster scores					
Social	Emotion and Eye Gaze	17	14	91	
	Communication	18	10	50	
	Gestures	19	14	91	
Speech	Sounds	18	12	75	
	Words	16	13	84	
Symbolic	Understanding	21	12	75	
	Object Use	17	11	63	
Composite scores					
	Social	54	14	91	
	Speech	34	12	75	
	Symbolic	38	12	75	
	TOTAL	126	114	83	

had a repeated up and down movement. It is important to notice that Abby distinguished these two different action schemes, and, therefore, we gave her credit for both actions.

HUNTER: 13 MONTHS

Comments on Sampling Procedures

Hunter used a combination of gestures, sounds, and some words to communicate. She displayed frequent gaze shifts but less shared positive affect than Camille or Abby. She used a broad range of communicative functions, and her sample included many nice examples of joint attention. The clinician and mother were very responsive to her communicative attempts and noticed and commented when Hunter directed their attention to objects. The clinician coached Hunter's mom effectively to ensure her active participation during the sample. The comprehension probes can be challenging to administer. Hunter's were not administered exactly as specified in the instructions for the sampling procedures. The clinician had too many of the play objects out and presented too many trials of object names and body parts. It is easy to present too many trials, and this error can be corrected when scoring the sample. The first four trials of object names and body parts and the first three trials of person names should be scored.

Comments on Scoring Decisions

Figure 6.3 shows a completed CSBS DP Behavior Sample: Scoring Worksheet for Hunter. Here are some examples of communicative acts used by her.

Behavior Regulation

#1: Hunter gave the wind-up toy to her mom to request her to wind it up.

#2: She said, "Uh uh," and took the Koosh duck back from the clinician to protest her putting it away.

#3: She reached to request more bubbles. (This was a distal gesture.)

#4: She said, "More," while giving the jar to her mom to request more cereal. (Her approximation of *more* ranged from *ma* to *mama* to *mamamama.*)

#5: Hunter said, "Mickey," while reaching toward the Mickey Mouse book to request that book from the choice of three books.

#6: She said, "Baba," while reaching toward the bottle to request the clinician to give her the bottle. (This was a distal gesture and a word approximation of *bottle.*)

Social Interaction

#1: She reached toward her mom and whined to request comfort. (Reaching could have been a contact gesture if she had touched her mom; however, this was a distal gesture because she did not.)

CSBS DP

CSBS DP Behavior Sample: Scoring Worksheet

Child's name: *Hunter*

Date completed: *5-28-00*

Date of birth: *4-5-99*

Chronological age[1]**:** *13 months*

[1] If child is 4 or more weeks premature, use corrected age. Calculate chronological age by subtracting Date of birth from Date the Behavior Sample was completed.

	1	2	3	4	5	6
Sampling Opportunity:	*Wind-up toy*	*Balloon*	*Bubbles*	*Jar*	*Books*	*Play*

COMMUNICATION SCALES (Score during Opportunities 1 to 6)

Emotion and Eye Gaze

	1	2	3	4	5	6
1. Gaze shifts	☒	☒	☒	☒	☒	☒
2. Shared positive affect	☐	☒	☒	☐	☐	☐
3. Gaze/point following		☒			☒	

Weighted Raw Score: Scale 1 [6] + Scale 2 [2] + Scale 3 _2_ × 3 [6] = **14**

Communication

	1	2	3	4	5	6
	✓✓	✓✓	✓✓	✓✓	✓✓	✓✓
4. Rate of communicating	0 1 2 (3+)	0 1 2 (3+)	0 1 2 (3+)	0 1 2 (3+)	0 1 2 (3+)	0 1 2 (3+)
5. Behavior regulation	☒	☒	☒	☒	☒	☒
6. Social interaction	☒	☐	☐	☒	☒	☐
7. Joint attention	☒	☒	☒	☐	☒	☒

Weighted Raw Score: Scale 4 _18_ ÷ 3 [6] + Scale 5 [6] + Scale 6 [3] + Scale 7 [5] = **20**

Gestures

8. Inventory of conventional gestures
check all that child uses:

☒ gives	☒ shows	☐ pushes/pulls away	☒ reaches
☒ points	☐ waves	☐ nods head	☐ shakes head

	1	2	3	4	5	6
9. Distal gestures	☒	☐	☒	☒	☐	☒

Weighted Raw Score: Scale 8 _4_ × 2 [8] + Scale 9 [4] = **12**

Sounds

	1	2	3	4	5	6
10. Syllables with consonants	☒	☒	☒	☒	☒	☒

11. Inventory of consonants
check all that child uses:

☒ /m/	☒ /n/	☒ /b/p/	☒ /d/t/	☒ /g/k/
☒ /w/	☐ /t/	☐ /y/	☒ /s/	☐ /sh/

Weighted Raw Score: Scale 10 [6] + Scale 11 _7_ × 2 [14] = **20**

Words

	1	2	3	4	5	6
12. Words	☒	☒	☒	☒	☒	☒

13. Inventory of words
write examples of words used:

1 *this (dis)*	2 *eyes*	3 *duck*	4 *baby*
5 *more (ma)*	6 *Mickey*	7 *bee (beebee)*	8 *baba*
9 *Mama*	10 *Mm (yum)*	11	12
13	14	15	16

	1	2	3	4	5	6
14. Word combinations	☐	☐	☐	☐	☐	☐

15. Inventory of word combinations
write examples of words combined:

1	2
3	4
5	6
7	8

Weighted Raw Score: Scale 12 [6] + Scale 13 _10_ ÷ 2 [5] + Scale 14 [0] + Scale 15 [0] = **11**

Figure 6.3. Completed CSBS DP Behavior Sample: Scoring Worksheet for Hunter.

SYMBOLIC BEHAVIOR SCALES (Score only during Opportunity 6 Play)

Understanding

16. Language comprehension

	1	2	3	4
object names:	cup	bottle	spoon	
person names:	Big Bird X	Mommy		
body parts:	ears	nose	teeth	eyes

(maximum of 3 raw score) (maximum of 2 raw score) (maximum of 3 raw score)

Weighted Raw Score: *Object names* 0 × 3 [0] + *Person names* 1 × 3 [3] + *Body parts* 0 × 3 [0] = 3

Object Use

17. Inventory of action schemes
check all that child uses:

☐ puts in [1]	☒ puts on [2]	☒ drinks with bottle [3]	☐ drinks with cup [4]	☒ hugs [5]	☒ kisses [6]
☒ feeds with utensil [7]	☐ feeds with bowl [8]	☒ stirs [9]	☒ scoops [10]	☐ pours [11]	other action: ☐ [12]

18. Action schemes toward other
write action numbers & agent's initials:

6 BB	7 BB	5 BB	3 BB		

19. Sequences action schemes
write action numbers:

10 + 7	9 + 7				

20. Stacks tower of blocks
circle highest number:

refuses, mouths, or bangs	tries but fails to stack	stacks	stacks	stacks	stacks
0	1	(2)	3	4	5

Weighted Raw Score: Scale 17 [7] + Scale 18 [4] + Scale 19 [2] + Scale 20 [2] = 15

CSBS DP Behavior Sample: Scoring Summary

		Weighted raw score	Standard score	Percentile rank	Concern
Cluster scores					
Social	Emotion and Eye Gaze	14	10	50	
	Communication	20	16	98	
	Gestures	12	10	50	
Speech	Sounds	20	17	99	
	Words	11	17	99	
Symbolic	Understanding	3	10	50	
	Object Use	15	17	99	
Composite scores					
	Social	46	11	63	
	Speech	31	17	99	
	Symbolic	18	12	75	
	TOTAL	95	125	95	

#4: She waved and said, "Bye-bye," to the dog figure as a greeting. (Although her hand went out of the range of the camera, this was counted as a distal gesture because it was clear that she was not touching an object; this was a verbal imitation of the clinician, and therefore, *bye-bye* was not counted as a word.)

Joint Attention

#1: Hunter tapped on the arm of the hook-on high chair and said, "Dis" (this) to draw attention to it.

#1: She said, "Eyes," first while looking at the clinician and then while pointing to the eye on the dog figure.

#2: Said, "Wewe," while reaching toward and touching the balloon after her mother blew it up. (This appeared to be an exclamatory comment to share the excitement, rather than a request for the balloon.)

#2: After pulling the Koosh duck out of the bag, she said, "Duck," along with other sounds and pointed to the face of the duck.

#2/3: She said, "Baby," in response to her mom asking, "What's that?" during the gaze/point following probe.

#6: She said, "Mmm," (approximation of *yum*) and looked at her mom while feeding herself with the spoon to comment on her play.

#6: She said, "Ah," and showed the spoon to the clinician.

During the symbolic play sample, Hunter used many different actions, some toward the Big Bird doll. Note that Hunter was credited for drinking from the bottle because she used this action at least two times. The first time, it was an imitation of the clinician, which did not count as an action scheme, but she used it again later when she fed the Big Bird doll with the bottle. Although many trials of language comprehension were presented, Hunter only demonstrated a correct response for identifying the Big Bird doll during the person names trial.

CHRISTI: 12 MONTHS

Comments on Sampling Procedures

Christi is a cooperative, cautious young child. The clinician paced the interaction slowly to follow Christi's temperament and style. This sample illustrates standard procedures with the exception of gaze/point following. The clinician presented the two trials in reverse order. The easier point to follow is behind the child and should be presented first.

Comments on Scoring Decisions

Figure 6.4 shows a completed CSBS DP Behavior Sample: Scoring Worksheet for Christi. Christi is preverbal and has a small repertoire of sounds and gestures.

CSBS DP

CSBS DP Behavior Sample: Scoring Worksheet

Child's name: Christi

Date completed: 4-27-02

Date of birth: 4-11-01

Chronological age[1]*:* 12 months

[1] If child is 4 or more weeks premature, use corrected age. Calculate chronological age by subtracting Date of birth from Date the Behavior Sample was completed.

Sampling Opportunity:	1	2	3	4	5	6
	Wind-up toy	*Balloon*	*Bubbles*	*Jar*	*Books*	*Play*

COMMUNICATION SCALES (Score during Opportunities 1 to 6)

Emotion and Eye Gaze

	1	2	3	4	5	6
1. Gaze shifts	X	X	X	X	☐	X
2. Shared positive affect	☐	X	X	☐	☐	X
3. Gaze/point following		X			X	

Weighted Raw Score: Scale 1 [5] + Scale 2 [3] + Scale 3 2 × 3 [6] = 14

Communication

	1	2	3	4	5	6
	✓✓	✓✓	✓✓	✓✓	✓✓	✓✓
4. Rate of communicating	0 1 2 3+	0 1 2 3+	0 1 2 3+	0 1 2 3+	0 1 2 3+	0 1 2 3+
5. Behavior regulation	X	X	X	X	X	X
6. Social interaction	X	X	☐	X	☐	X
7. Joint attention	X	X	X	☐	X	☐

Weighted Raw Score: Scale 4 18 ÷ 3 [6] + Scale 5 [6] + Scale 6 [4] + Scale 7 [4] = 20

Gestures

8. Inventory of conventional gestures *check all that child uses:*

X gives	X shows	X pushes/pulls away	X reaches
X points	X waves	☐ nods head	☐ shakes head

	1	2	3	4	5	6
9. Distal gestures	X	X	X	X	X	X

Weighted Raw Score: Scale 8 6 × 2 [12] + Scale 9 [6] = 18

Sounds

	1	2	3	4	5	6
10. Syllables with consonants	☐	X	☐	☐	☐	☐

11. Inventory of consonants *check all that child uses:*

☐ /m/	☐ /n/	☐ /blp/	X /dlt/	☐ /glk/
☐ /w/	☐ /t/	☐ /y/	☐ /s/	☐ /sh/

Weighted Raw Score: Scale 10 [1] + Scale 11 1 × 2 [2] = 3

Words

	1	2	3	4	5	6
12. Words	☐	☐	☐	☐	☐	☐

13. Inventory of words *write examples of words used:*

1	2	3	4
5	6	7	8
9	10	11	12
13	14	15	16

	1	2	3	4	5	6
14. Word combinations	☐	☐	☐	☐	☐	☐

15. Inventory of word combinations *write examples of words combined:*

1	2
3	4
5	6
7	8

Weighted Raw Score: Scale 12 [0] + Scale 13 ____ ÷ 2 [0] + Scale 14 [0] + Scale 15 [0] = 0

Figure 6.4. Completed CSBS DP Behavior Sample: Scoring Worksheet for Christi.

SYMBOLIC BEHAVIOR SCALES (Score only during Opportunity 6 Play)

Understanding

16. Language comprehension

object names:	cup [1]	spoon [2]	X bottle [3]	X bowl [4]
person names:	Mommy [1]	Big Bird [2]	[3]	
body parts:	eyes [1]	hands [2]	[3]	[4]

(maximum of 3 raw score) (maximum of 2 raw score) (maximum of 3 raw score)

Weighted Raw Score: *Object names* 2 × 3 [6] + *Person names* 0 × 3 [0] + *Body parts* 0 × 3 [0] = [6]

Object Use

17. Inventory of action schemes
check all that child uses:

☒ puts in [1]	❐ puts on [2]	❐ drinks with bottle [3]	❐ drinks with cup [4]	❐ hugs [5]	❐ kisses [6]
☒ feeds with utensil [7]	❐ feeds with bowl [8]	❐ stirs [9]	❐ scoops [10]	☒ pours [11]	other action: ❐ [12]

18. Action schemes toward other
write action numbers & agent's initials:

7 Cl					

19. Sequences action schemes
write action numbers:

11 + 7					

20. Stacks tower of blocks
circle highest number:

refuses, mouths, or bangs	tries but fails to stack	stacks	stacks	stacks	stacks
0	1	2	3	4	5

Weighted Raw Score: Scale 17 [3] + Scale 18 [1] + Scale 19 [1] + Scale 20 [2] = [7]

CSBS DP

CSBS DP Behavior Sample: Scoring Summary

		Weighted raw score	Standard score	Percentile rank	Concern
Cluster scores					
Social	Emotion and Eye Gaze	14	10	50	
	Communication	20	16	98	
	Gestures	18	16	98	
Speech	Sounds	3	7	16	
	Words	0	10	50	
Symbolic	Understanding	6	12	75	
	Object Use	7	9	37	
Composite scores					
	Social	52	15	95	
	Speech	3	8	25	
	Symbolic	13	11	63	
TOTAL		68	102	55	

Because of this fact, her sample is relatively easy to score. She used the consonants /m/, /b/, and /w/ during the sample, but she did not use them within communicative acts, and therefore, they were not counted as consonants in her inventory. She readily used distal gestures throughout the sample. Christi had fewer gaze shifts and shared positive affect than the previous children. During Opportunity 1, she had a few clear gaze shifts and at one point looked at the clinician with a smirk, but this was not counted as shared positive affect because it was not clear enough to be considered a smile. In contrast, during Opportunity 2 she had a clear example of shared positive affect after the second time the balloon flew away; she looked at her mom, smiled, laughed, and looked over to the clinician. During Opportunity 3, she displayed a gaze shift when she held the jar of bubbles and gave it to her mom to open it because she looked at the jar, looked up at her mom, and looked back at the jar. Then, she smiled but did not share positive affect. Next, she popped bubbles and smiled, looked at her mom, and laughed softly. This action was counted as shared positive affect. She displayed a gaze shift during Opportunity 4 as she was putting the foot-shaped teether back in the bag and looked at the bag, then looked at her mother, and back at the bag. During Opportunity 6, she displayed a clear gaze shift and shared positive affect while stacking the blocks. Christi was able to follow the gaze and point of the clinician by turning her head for both gaze/point following probes. Remember that only a 45 degree turn is needed to be credited.

Christi seemed very interested in the books. Just before she was offered three books, Christi looked at the bag of toys and vocalized /ba/. This was not counted as a communicative act because it was not directed. While examining the first book, she turned the pages but did not shift gaze to a person. She vocalized /wawa/ but this was not a communicative act because it was not directed to a person. Here are some good examples of communicative acts used by Christi:

Behavior Regulation

#1: Christi pointed to the toy bag on the floor to request a toy. (This was counted as a distal gesture.)

#2: She gave the balloon to her mom to request her to blow it up.

#2: She gave the balloon to her mom and vocalized /dada/ in response to her mom saying, "You want me to do it again?"

#2: She pushed away Mr. Potato Head to protest and indicated she didn't want him.

#3: Christi gave the jar of bubbles to her mom to request blowing bubbles.

#4: She tapped the lid of the jar that her mom was holding and vocalized /a a/ to request more Cheerios.

#4: She gave the foot-shaped teether to her mom after taking it out of the bag to have her mom hold it. (It was believed that this was a request for action because she abandoned attention to the teether as soon as she gave it to her mom and shifted her attention back to the bag in front of her.)

#6: She gave the cup to her mom and vocalized /dada/ to request her mom to hold the cup.

Social Interaction

#2: She waved across the room to greet Mr. Potato Head and then reached toward her mom and fussed to request comfort. (It was believed that this wave was a greeting because Christi's focus remained on Mr. Potato Head and then shifted to her mom. When Christi's mom brought Mr. Potato Head to her, he was not what she wanted, and she continued waving.)

#4: Christi reached toward her mom and vocalized /a/ to request comfort.

Joint Attention

#1: She showed the Big Bird/Little Bird figure to the clinician after pulling him out of the bag.

#1: She gave the Big Bird/Little Bird figure to her mom to get her to look at him and share attention on him. (It was felt that this give was a comment because the focus of her attention remained on the Big Bird figure while her mom examined it, and she wanted the figure back.)

#2: She showed and then gave the hand-shaped teether to the clinician to share attention on it. (Again, it was felt the this was for joint attention because Christi's attention stayed on the teether, and she wanted it back.)

#3 She showed and then gave the dog to her mom to share attention on it. (Again, her focus of attention was on the dog until her mom gave it back.)

Unclear

#1: Waved to Mr. Potato Head, who was on a shelf out of reach. It was unclear at this point whether Christi was greeting Mr. Potato Head or requesting her mom to get him. This act can be counted as a distal gesture and a wave and can be counted toward her rate of communicating but would not count as a communicative function. Because Christi displayed all three functions in other acts during this opportunity, the unclear function does not affect her score.

PATRICK "THOMAS": 13 MONTHS

Comments on Sampling Procedures

Thomas was active and energetic. The pace of the sample was upbeat and followed his interest. Notice that during the balloon temptation, Thomas bit the balloon before the clinician had a chance to move it away from his mouth, and it broke. Because Thomas is so boisterous, he was not frightened. If possible, it is best to prevent a child from biting the balloon; however, if this event can't be prevented and the balloon breaks, it is imperative that the clinician immediately find all of the pieces of the balloon and remove them so that the child cannot have access to broken pieces of the balloon. We have found that the balloon opportunity can stimulate interesting affect and communication, but it is important to recognize the perils of balloons around young children and to take serious precautions.

Comments on Scoring Decisions

Figure 6.5 shows a completed CSBS DP Behavior Sample: Scoring Worksheet for Thomas. He displayed frequent gaze shifts and shared positive affect. Many of his vocalizations during the sample were not part of communicative acts and were not counted. It is important to notice whether he directed them to an adult. A big issue in scoring Thomas's sample was whether his behavior met the criteria for a communicative act. During the first opportunity, he shook the wind-up toy and looked at his mom. This was not considered to be a communicative act because his focus of attention shifted away so quickly there was no evidence of a communicative goal or purpose. When he pulled the dog out of the bag, he said, "Ga," but did not direct this response with eye gaze or a gesture. He banged the dog on the table and said, "Wawa"; this response was not considered a communicative act because it was not directed to an adult. The following are some good examples of communicative acts used by Thomas:

Behavior Regulation

#1: Thomas gave the wind-up toy to the clinician to request her to wind it up.

#2: He gave the balloon to the clinician and said, "Help."

#2: He reached toward the bag after he pulled out the Big Bird figure from the bag.

#4: He gave the jar to the clinician and said, "Didi," to request more Cheerios.

Social Interaction

#2: Thomas waved to the Big Bird doll to greet it as it was being removed.

#5: He held the book over his head, said, "Peek," then removed it and looked at the clinician to draw attention to himself for Peekaboo.

Joint Attention

#1: He showed the jar of bubbles to the clinician by shaking it to get her attention.

#3: He said, "Ish," while looking at the picture on the wall and then looking at the clinician; then he repeated this sequence to share attention on the picture.

#6: After his mom fed him with a spoon, Thomas vocalized, "Oo," and looked at his mom to share the moment. Then, he fed his mom with a spoon.

CSBS DP

CSBS DP Behavior Sample: Scoring Worksheet

Child's name: Patrick "Thomas"

Date completed: 9-3-01

Date of birth: 7-24-00

Chronological age[1]: 13 months

[1] If child is 4 or more weeks premature, use corrected age. Calculate chronological age by subtracting Date of birth from Date the Behavior Sample was completed.

Sampling Opportunity:	1 Wind-up toy	2 Balloon	3 Bubbles	4 Jar	5 Books	6 Play

COMMUNICATION SCALES (Score during Opportunities 1 to 6)

Emotion and Eye Gaze

	1	2	3	4	5	6
1. Gaze shifts	☒	☒	☒	☒	☒	☒
2. Shared positive affect	☒	☐	☐	☐	☒	☒
3. Gaze/point following		☒			☒	

Weighted Raw Score: Scale 1 [6] + Scale 2 [3] + Scale 3 2 × 3 [6] = **15**

Communication

	1	2	3	4	5	6
4. Rate of communicating	✓ 0 1 2 3+	✓✓ 0 1 2 3+	✓✓ 0 1 2 3+	✓✓ 0 1 2 3+	✓✓ 0 1 2 3+	✓ 0 1 2 3+
5. Behavior regulation	☒	☒	☒	☒	☐	☐
6. Social interaction	☐	☒	☐	☐	☒	☐
7. Joint attention	☐	☐	☒	☒	☐	☒

Weighted Raw Score: Scale 4 15 ÷ 3 [5] + Scale 5 [4] + Scale 6 [2] + Scale 7 [3] = **14**

Gestures

8. Inventory of conventional gestures *check all that child uses:*

☒ gives	☒ shows	☒ pushes/pulls away	☒ reaches
☒ points	☒ waves	☐ nods head	☐ shakes head

	1	2	3	4	5	6
9. Distal gestures	☐	☒	☐	☒	☐	☐

Weighted Raw Score: Scale 8 6 × 2 [12] + Scale 9 [2] = **14**

Sounds

	1	2	3	4	5	6
10. Syllables with consonants	☐	☒	☒	☒	☒	☐

11. Inventory of consonants *check all that child uses:*

☐ /m/	☐ /n/	☒ /blp/	☒ /dlt/	☐ /glk/
☐ /w/	☐ /t/	☐ /y/	☐ /s/	☐ /sh/

Weighted Raw Score: Scale 10 [4] + Scale 11 2 × 2 [4] = **8**

Words

	1	2	3	4	5	6
12. Words	☐	☒	☐	☐	☐	☐

13. Inventory of words *write examples of words used:*

help 1	2	3	4
5	6	7	8
9	10	11	12
13	14	15	16

	1	2	3	4	5	6
14. Word combinations	☐	☐	☐	☐	☐	☐

15. Inventory of word combinations *write examples of words combined:*

1	2
3	4
5	6
7	8

Weighted Raw Score: Scale 12 [1] + Scale 13 1 ÷ 2 [1] + Scale 14 [0] + Scale 15 [0] = **2**

Figure 6.5. Completed CSBS DP Behavior Sample: Scoring Worksheet for Patrick "Thomas."

SYMBOLIC BEHAVIOR SCALES (Score only during Opportunity 6 Play)

Understanding

16. Language comprehension

object names:	cup [1]	bottle [2]	spoon [3]	[4]
person names:	Mommy [1]	[2]	[3]	
body parts:	eyes [1]	hands [2]	[3]	[4]

(maximum of 3 raw score) (maximum of 2 raw score) (maximum of 3 raw score)

Weighted Raw Score: *Object names* 0 × 3 [0] + *Person names* 0 × 3 [0] + *Body parts* 0 × 3 [0] = 0

Object Use

17. Inventory of action schemes

check all that child uses:

☒ puts in [1]	☐ puts on [2]	☒ drinks with bottle [3]	☐ drinks with cup [4]	☒ hugs [5]	☐ kisses [6]
☒ feeds with utensil [7]	☐ feeds with bowl [8]	☒ stirs [9]	☐ scoops [10]	☐ pours [11]	other action: ☐ [12]

18. Action schemes toward other

write action numbers & agent's initials:

5 BB	7 Mom	7 BB			

19. Sequences action schemes

write action numbers:

20. Stacks tower of blocks

circle highest number:

refuses, mouths, or bangs	tries but fails to stack	stacks	stacks	stacks	stacks
0	1	2	3	4	5

Weighted Raw Score: Scale 17 [5] + Scale 18 [3] + Scale 19 [0] + Scale 20 [2] = 10

CSBS DP™ CSBS DP Behavior Sample: Scoring Summary

		Weighted raw score	Standard score	Percentile rank	Concern
Cluster scores					
Social	Emotion and Eye Gaze	15	11	63	
	Communication	14	9	37	
	Gestures	14	11	63	
Speech	Sounds	8	10	50	
	Words	2	12	75	
Symbolic	Understanding	0	8	25	
	Object Use	10	12	75	
Composite scores					
	Social	43	10	50	
	Speech	10	10	50	
	Symbolic	10	9	37	
	TOTAL	63	97	42	

KYLA: 12 MONTHS

Comments on Sampling Procedures

Kyla used a combination of gestures, sounds, and some words to communicate. She displayed very frequent gaze shifts and shared positive affect. She used a broad range of communicative functions, and her sample included many nice examples of joint attention. The clinician did an excellent job responding to and expanding on her many communicative acts. The sample was longer than needed because for each opportunity she displayed many instances of some types of communicative acts. The clinician presented too many trials of object names for the language comprehension probes, but this can be corrected by scoring the first four trials of object names that were not botched (see Comments on Scoring Decisions).

Comments on Scoring Decisions

Figure 6.6 shows a completed CSBS DP Behavior Sample: Scoring Worksheet for Kyla. Here are some good examples of communicative acts she used:

Behavior Regulation

#1: Kyla gave the wind-up toy to the clinician to request her to wind it up.

#2: She pushed the balloon away and cried to protest.

#3: She gave the jar of bubbles to her mom and said, "O," to request her to open it.

#4: She gave the jar of Cheerios to her mom and said, "Dit," to request her to open the jar.

#4: She reached toward the empty bag of toys and said, "Uh," to request it.

#5: Kyla gave the book to her mom and said, "Da," to request her to help open the book.

Social Interaction

#1: She banged the wind-up toy in a turn-taking game to draw attention to herself. (It is believed that this action was social interaction because the focus of attention was on the interaction rather than on the object.)

#3: She banged and vocalized with the dog figure in a turn-taking game with the clinician.

#4: She looked at her mom and vocalized to call her attention.

#5: Kyla raised her arms while vocalizing, "Dodo," smiling, and looking at the clinician to show off.

CSBS DP

CSBS DP Behavior Sample: Scoring Worksheet

Child's name: *Kyla*

Date completed: *4-25-01*

Date of birth: *4-10-00*

Chronological age[1]**:** *12 months*

[1] If child is 4 or more weeks premature, use corrected age. Calculate chronological age by subtracting Date of birth from Date the Behavior Sample was completed.

	1	2	3	4	5	6
Sampling Opportunity:	*Wind-up toy*	*Balloon*	*Bubbles*	*Jar*	*Books*	*Play*

COMMUNICATION SCALES (Score during Opportunities 1 to 6)

Emotion and Eye Gaze

	1	2	3	4	5	6
1. Gaze shifts	☒	☒	☒	☒	☒	☒
2. Shared positive affect	☒	☒	☒	☒	☒	☒
3. Gaze/point following		☒			☒	

Weighted Raw Score: Scale 1 [6] + Scale 2 [6] + Scale 3 _2_ × 3 [6] = **18**

Communication

	1	2	3	4	5	6
4. Rate of communicating	✓✓ 0 1 2 3+	✓✓ 0 1 2 3+	✓✓ 0 1 2 3+	✓✓ 0 1 2 3+	✓✓ 0 1 2 3+	✓✓ 0 1 2 3+
5. Behavior regulation	☒	☒	☒	☒	☒	☒
6. Social interaction	☒	☐	☒	☒	☒	☐
7. Joint attention	☒	☒	☒	☒	☒	☒

Weighted Raw Score: Scale 4 _18_ ÷ 3 [6] + Scale 5 [6] + Scale 6 [4] + Scale 7 [6] = **22**

Gestures

8. Inventory of conventional gestures
check all that child uses:

☒ gives	☒ shows	☒ pushes/pulls away	☒ reaches
☒ points	☐ waves	☐ nods head	☐ shakes head

	1	2	3	4	5	6
9. Distal gestures	☐	☒	☒	☒	☒	☒

Weighted Raw Score: Scale 8 _5_ × 2 [10] + Scale 9 [5] = **15**

Sounds

	1	2	3	4	5	6
10. Syllables with consonants	☒	☒	☒	☒	☒	☒

11. Inventory of consonants
check all that child uses:

☐ /m/	☐ /n/	☒ /b/p/	☒ /d/t/	☐ /g/k/
☒ /w/	☐ /t/	☒ /y/	☐ /s/	☐ /sh/

Weighted Raw Score: Scale 10 [6] + Scale 11 _4_ × 2 [8] = **14**

Words

	1	2	3	4	5	6
12. Words	☐	☐	☒	☐	☒	☐

13. Inventory of words
write examples of words used:

doggie (dado) 1	2	3	4
5	6	7	8
9	10	11	12
13	14	15	16

	1	2	3	4	5	6
14. Word combinations	☐	☐	☐	☐	☐	☐

15. Inventory of word combinations
write examples of words combined:

1	2
3	4
5	6
7	8

Weighted Raw Score: Scale 12 [2] + Scale 13 _1_ ÷ 2 [1] + Scale 14 [0] + Scale 15 [0] = **3**

Figure 6.6. Completed CSBS DP Behavior Sample: Scoring Worksheet for Kyla.

SYMBOLIC BEHAVIOR SCALES (Score only during Opportunity 6 Play)

Understanding

16. Language comprehension

object names:	spoon [1]	X bottle [2]	cup [3]	[4]
person names:	X Mommy [1]	X Big Bird [2]	[3]	
body parts:	X hands [1]	knees [2]	X hair [3]	eyes [4]

(maximum of 3 raw score) (maximum of 2 raw score) (maximum of 3 raw score)

Weighted Raw Score: *Object names* 2 × 3 [6] + *Person names* 2 × 3 [6] + *Body parts* 2 × 3 [6] = [18]

Object Use

17. Inventory of action schemes
check all that child uses:

☒ puts in [1]	☒ puts on [2]	☒ drinks with bottle [3]	☐ drinks with cup [4]	☒ hugs [5]	☐ kisses [6]
☒ feeds with utensil [7]	☐ feeds with bowl [8]	☒ stirs [9]	☐ scoops [10]	☐ pours [11]	other action: ☐ [12]

18. Action schemes toward other
write action numbers & agent's initials:

5 BB	3 BB	7 BB			

19. Sequences action schemes
write action numbers:

20. Stacks tower of blocks
circle highest number:

refuses, mouths, or bangs	tries but fails to stack	stacks	stacks	stacks	stacks
0	1	2	3	4	5

Weighted Raw Score: Scale 17 [6] + Scale 18 [3] + Scale 19 [0] + Scale 20 [1] = [10]

CSBS DP™

CSBS DP Behavior Sample: Scoring Summary

		Weighted raw score	Standard score	Percentile rank	Concern
Cluster scores					
Social	Emotion and Eye Gaze	18	17	99	
	Communication	22	17	99	
	Gestures	15	12	75	
Speech	Sounds	14	13	84	
	Words	3	13	84	
Symbolic	Understanding	18	15	95	
	Object Use	10	12	75	
Composite scores					
	Social	55	17	99	
	Speech	17	13	84	
	Symbolic	28	15	95	
	TOTAL	100	130	98	

Joint Attention

#1: She showed the wind-up toy to the clinician and said, "Dootdo," to draw her attention to it.

#1: She showed (shook) the wind-up toy to her mom and squealed after it deactivated to draw attention to it and share affect.

#2: She pointed to the picture on the wall after the clinician pointed and looked at the clinician to share attention on the picture. (This was a distal gesture.)

#3: She banged the dog figure on the table after taking it out of the bag and said, "Dododo, dado," (Kyla's word approximation for doggie) and looked at the clinician to draw the clinician's attention to it.

#4: She held up the empty bag of toys to show the clinician it was empty and vocalized, "Do ba."

#5: She pointed to a picture of a fox in the book, looked at the clinician and her mom, and said, "Dado."

Because there were too many trials of body parts presented during the language comprehension probes, score the first four trials that were not botched. The first trial was *hands*, and Kyla responded correctly. The second trial was *knees*, and she responded incorrectly. (It is recommended that you avoid a body part such as knees because it is later emerging, and the body part was not visible to Kyla; however, her mom had suggested it as one that she knew.) The next trial was *nose*, but this trial was botched because Kyla was touching her nose as the clinician said it. The following trial was *hair*, and she responded correctly. The trial after that was *ears*, but this trial was botched because Kyla was touching her *ears* as the clinician said it. The next trial was *eyes*, and she did not correctly identify them. The four trials recorded on the worksheet were the first four that were not botched, which were *hands*, *knees*, *hair*, and *eyes*. Kyla received credit for two of the four.

The clinician then proceeded to have Kyla identify body parts with her mom. These trials were not scored because they exceeded the number that should be presented. What is clear from Kyla's attempts to identify body parts on herself and her mother is that this skill is emerging. Her score of 2 out of 4 trials reflects that.

TECHNICAL CHARACTERISTICS 7

This chapter describes the technical characteristics for each of the three components of the CSBS DP—the CSBS DP Infant-Toddler Checklist, the CSBS DP Caregiver Questionnaire, and the CSBS DP Behavior Sample. The first part of this chapter addresses the characteristics of the sample used for standardization. The remainder of the chapter examines data on the reliability and validity of the CSBS DP.

STANDARDIZATION

The CSBS DP was developed and field-tested with children younger than 24 months of age. The difficulty in evaluating young children with existing tests made clear the need for an instrument such as the CSBS DP. As this instrument was developed and administered over time, scales that proved to be less reliable or discriminating were discarded or revised. Other measures shown by research or clinical observation to discriminate between children with more severe versus less severe delays were added. See Chapter 2 for research used as the basis for development of the CSBS DP.

The Preliminary Research Edition of the CSBS DP (Wetherby & Prizant, 1998) was standardized from 1997 to 2000. The standardization consisted of collecting Infant-Toddler Checklists, Caregiver Questionnaires, and Behavior Samples from children and scoring each to derive norms. A parent or other caregiver knowledgeable about the child completed the CSBS DP Infant-Toddler Checklists and the CSBS DP Caregiver Questionnaires. A parent or caregiver was present during the collection of the CSBS DP Behavior Sample, which was recorded on videotape for later analysis. The videotaped Behavior Samples were scored by a group of raters trained by the first author. The raters were certified speech-language pathologists or graduate students in speech-language pathology. Training consisted of 1) the author presenting to the group an overview of each communication and symbolic parameter to be rated, 2) each rater viewing and rating each of the six videotaped Behavior Samples included in the CSBS DP kit, and 3) the author and raters discussing their ratings. Before raters began rating tapes for the normative study, they rated two additional tapes to calibrate with the ratings of the experienced rater.

Standardization Sample

A total of 2,188 Infant-Toddler Checklists, 790 Caregiver Questionnaires, and 337 Behavior Samples were included in the standardization sample. Children were recruited for the standardization sample from a total of eight sites in the United States and two sites in Canada; however, the majority of children in the standardization sample were recruited from the Tallahassee, Florida, region; therefore, although the standardization sample is large, it is not a nationally representative sample. Sources for recruiting children included doctor offices, child care centers, and health fairs or other community events and sites regularly attended by families of young children. Children with known developmental delays or who qualified for Part C early intervention services were excluded from the standardization sample but were included in some validation studies reported in this chapter. Because of the extent of the under-identification of children with developmental delays from birth to 24 months of age, it is presumed that at least 10% of the standardization sample has developmental delays or disabilities, although children with severe disabilities are likely not included in this sample.

The children ranged in age from 6 to 24 months for the CSBS DP Infant-Toddler Checklist and CSBS DP Caregiver Questionnaire and from 12 to 24 months for the CSBS DP Behavior Sample. Because it was expected that the CSBS DP would be used more than once in evaluating children's communication and symbolic behavior over the course of several months, approximately 15% of the standardization sample was retested within an average of 2–3 months after the initial administration. These second administrations were included in the normative scores because, as Angoff (1971) pointed out, they increase the relevance of the norms to their intended use and reduce the error that would be associated with estimates of developmental improvement based on different children at different ages. This method of data collection made it possible to create data sets that include both cross-sectional and longitudinal data. (For more detail on the retested children, see the discussion of stability later in this chapter.)

The standardization sample is described in Tables 7.1–7.6 for several important demographic variables, including child's age at CSBS DP administration (Table 7.1), gender (Table 7.2), race (Table 7.3), Hispanic origin (Table 7.4), and parent age and education (Tables 7.5 and 7.6).

Age

Table 7.1 shows the number of children and the percentage of the total standardization sample at each age interval for the CSBS DP Infant-Toddler Checklist, CSBS DP Caregiver Questionnaire, and CSBS DP Behavior Sample. The children are grouped according to age in intervals that correspond with the norms presented in the Appendixes. For the Infant-Toddler Checklist, norms are presented in 1-month intervals from 6 to 24 months of age. For the Caregiver Questionnaire, norms are presented in 2-month intervals, with the exception of 12 months of age, which is presented as a single-month interval because of the larger sample size at that age. For the Behavior Sample, norms are presented in 3-month intervals from 12 to 20 months of age, and a 4-month interval from 21 to 24 months of age. As can be seen, most of the age intervals include at least 60 children and many include more than 100 children. Only one interval includes less than 30 children (i.e., 6–7 months for the CSBS DP Caregiver Questionnaire); therefore, caution should be taken in using the norms for the Caregiver Questionnaire for children younger than 8 months of age.

Gender

Table 7.2 shows the number of children by gender for the Infant-Toddler Checklist, Caregiver Questionnaire, and Behavior Sample. This table shows an almost equal

Table 7.1. Children in the standardization sample, by age in months

Infant-Toddler Checklist			Caregiver Questionnaire			Behavior Sample		
Age (months)	*n*	Percent of total	Age (months)	*n*	Percent of total	Age (months)	*n*	Percent of total
6	50	2.3	6–7	12	1.5	12–14	82	24.3
7	42	1.9	8–9	47	5.9	15–17	76	22.6
8	77	3.5	10–11	53	6.7	18–20	76	22.6
9	126	5.8	12	71	9.0	21–24	103	30.6
10	86	3.9	13–14	107	13.5	**Total**	**337**	**100.0**
11	312	14.3	15–16	129	16.3			
12	296	13.5	17–18	114	14.4			
13	121	5.5	19–20	113	14.3			
14	128	5.9	21–22	89	11.3			
15	174	8.0	23–24	55	7.0			
16	98	4.5	**Total**	**790**	**100.0**			
17	99	4.5						
18	133	6.1						
19	107	4.9						
20	84	3.8						
21	87	4.0						
22	82	3.7						
23	50	2.3						
24	36	1.6						
Total	**2188**	**100.0**						

balance of males and females for the CSBS DP Infant-Toddler Checklist and CSBS DP Behavior Sample, and slightly more males represented in the CSBS DP Caregiver Questionnaire.

Race and Ethnicity

Tables 7.3 and 7.4 show the number and percentage of children in the standardization sample by race and Hispanic origin, respectively, for the Infant-Toddler Checklist, Caregiver Questionnaire, and Behavior Sample. The majority of children in the standardization sample for all three components were Caucasian; however, a substantial number of African American children were included in the standardization sample for the Infant-Toddler Checklist and Caregiver Questionnaire, well above the percentage in the U.S. population, based on 2000 population estimates from the U.S. Census Bureau. The reason that the percentage of African American children is so high for the Infant-Toddler Checklist and Caregiver Questionnaire is that a large proportion of the sample was drawn from the Tallahassee region and approximately one fourth of the population in that region is African American. A lower percentage of African American children were included in the standardization sample for the Behavior Sample, which reflects the fact that the Tallahassee region was a smaller proportion of the standardization sample for the CSBS DP Behavior Sample and that there was difficulty recruiting African American families for the face-to-face evaluation. Thus, African American

Table 7.2. Children in the standardization sample, by gender

	Infant-Toddler Checklist		Caregiver Questionnaire		Behavior Sample	
Gender	*n*	Percent of total	*n*	Percent of total	*n*	Percent of total
Female	1090	49.8	375	47.5	165	49.0
Male	1098	50.2	415	52.5	172	51.0
Total	**2188**	**100.0**	**790.0**	**100.0**	**337.0**	**100.0**

Table 7.3. Children in the standardization sample, by race

U.S. population[a]		Infant-Toddler Checklist		Caregiver Questionnaire		Behavior Sample	
Race	Percent of total	*n*	Percent of total	*n*	Percent of total	*n*	Percent of total
White	75.1	1504	71.5	615	78.2	288	87.0
Black	12.3	483	23.0	128	16.3	30	9.1
Asian	3.6	61	2.9	18	2.3	10	3.0
Other	8.9	56	2.7	25	3.2	3	0.9
Total	**100.0**	**2104**	**100.0**	**786**	**100.0**	**331**	**100.0**

[a]Based on 2000 U.S. Census Bureau figures

Table 7.4. Children in the standardization sample, by Hispanic origin

U.S. population[a]		Infant-Toddler Checklist		Caregiver Questionnaire		Behavior Sample	
Hispanic	Percent of total	*n*	Percent of total	*n*	Percent of total	*n*	Percent of total
Yes	12.5	120	5.5	49	6.2	21	6.2
No	87.5	2068	94.5	741	93.8	316	93.8
Total	**100.0**	**2188**	**100.0**	**790**	**100.0**	**337**	**100.0**

[a]Based on 2000 U.S. Census Bureau figures

children are over-represented in the standardization samples for the Infant-Toddler Checklist and Caregiver Questionnaire and under-represented in the standardization sample for the Behavior Sample. The proportion of children in the standardization sample who were of Hispanic origin is below that represented on average in the United States, based on the 2000 Census data. The proportions reported in Tables 7.3 and 7.4 indicate that the standardization sample is a diverse group but that it does not adequately represent the diversity of the U.S. population for the CSBS DP Behavior Sample. *Therefore, caution should be taken when using the CSBS DP Behavior Sample norms with minority populations.*

Parent Age and Education

Table 7.5 shows the average age and amount of education for parents of children in the standardization sample for the Infant-Toddler Checklist, Caregiver Questionnaire, and Behavior Sample because these variables are strongly indicative of socio-

Table 7.5. Parent's age at childbirth and years of education for children in standardization sample

	Infant-Toddler Checklist	Caregiver Questionnaire	Behavior Sample
Mother's age			
Mean	29.3	30.3	31.0
Standard deviation	6.0	6.0	5.9
Range	12.6–45.5	12.6–42.9	18–42.9
Father's age			
Mean	31.7	32.8	33.6
Standard deviation	7.1	6.9	6.5
Range	14.3–60.9	14.3–50.9	20.8–50.9
Mother's education			
Mean	14.7	15.0	15.2
Standard deviation	2.2	2.2	2.3
Range	8–21	8–21	11–20
Father's education			
Mean	14.6	14.8	15.1
Standard deviation	2.6	2.6	2.6
Range	8–22	9–22	9–21

economic class. Table 7.5 reports the average ages of the mother and father at the time of the child's birth in years. It also reports the average number of years of education for the mother and father, ranging from 8, indicating completion of eighth grade, to 22, indicating completion of twelfth grade plus 4 years of undergraduate school and 6 years of graduate or medical school.

Table 7.6 shows the amount of education for the mothers and fathers of children in the standardization sample for the Infant-Toddler Checklist, Caregiver Questionnaire, and Behavior Sample in relation to the 2000 U.S. Census Bureau figures, based on completion of less than high school, high school, some college, and a college degree. The proportions reported in Table 7.6 indicate that the education level of the parents of children in the standardization sample is above the national average.

The demographic information reported in Tables 7.5 and 7.6 suggests that the socioeconomic level of these families is above the national average. *Therefore, caution should be taken when using the norms for the CSBS DP with parents who have low education levels, particularly those who have not completed high school.*

DEVELOPMENT OF NORMATIVE SCORES

The development of norms required a balance of concern for several elements of CSBS DP construction, including the wide variety of communication and symbolic behavior parameters rated, the uneven growth of these parameters within the age range of the standardization sample, the variability with the obtained sample, and the intended use of the CSBS DP norms in comparing observed and expected performance not only for children within but also outside the age range of the standardization group. The considerable differences among the ranges of possible raw scores on items on the CSBS DP Caregiver Questionnaire and CSBS DP Behavior Sample required a method for adjusting scores within cluster areas to be comparable with

Table 7.6. Children in the standardization sample, by parent's education

	U.S. population[a]	Infant-Toddler Checklist		Caregiver Questionnaire		Behavior Sample	
	Percent of total	*n*	Percent of total	*n*	Percent of total	*n*	Percent of total
Mother's education							
Some high school or less	15.0	79	3.8	35	4.5	2	0.6
High school diploma	29.2	444	21.4	140	17.9	37	11.3
Some college	34.4	473	22.8	144	18.4	60	18.3
College degree	21.5	1082	52.1	463	59.2	229	69.8
Total	**100.0**	**2078**	**100.0**	**782**	**100.0**	**328**	**100.0**
Father's education							
Some high school or less	18.4	82	4.2	41	5.4	10	3.1
High school diploma	31.8	553	28.0	185	24.5	52	16.0
Some college	30.6	373	18.9	122	16.2	57	17.5
College degree	19.2	965	48.9	407	53.9	206	63.4
Total	**100.0**	**1973**	**100.0**	**755**	**100.0**	**325**	**100.0**

[a]Based on 2000 U.S. Census Bureau figures for 18- to 34-year-olds

each other. This was done by weighting items using a multiplication or division factor, as described in the scoring instructions in Chapter 4 for the Caregiver Questionnaire and Chapter 5 for the Behavior Sample.

The first step was to generate scores that would aid in interpretation of various patterns of performance on related items. These scores, called *cluster scores*, are based on summing the raw scores for meaningful combinations of items. The CSBS DP has seven clusters for each of the components, based on the original conceptual model for the CSBS. These clusters were named for simplicity but correspond with the CSBS clusters as follows, with the cluster name from the CSBS in parentheses:

1. Emotion and Eye Gaze (Social-Affective Signaling)
2. Communication (Communicative Functions and Reciprocity)
3. Gestures (Gestural Communicative Means)
4. Sounds (Vocal Communicative Means)
5. Words (Verbal Communicative Means)
6. Understanding (Symbolic Behavior)
7. Object Use (Symbolic Behavior)

The cluster scores were calculated using the raw scores for the CSBS DP Infant-Toddler Checklist and the weighted raw scores for the CSBS DP Caregiver Questionnaire and CSBS DP Behavior Sample. Because the Infant-Toddler Checklist has a small number of items and range of scores within each cluster, norms were not created at the level of the cluster scores for the Infant-Toddler Checklist. For the Caregiver Questionnaire and Behavior Sample, the resulting sum for each combination of items was then obtained for each child in the standardization sample, and a frequency distribution for each of the combined raw scores or weighted raw scores was obtained for each age interval. Percentile ranks derived from each frequency distribution were then converted, using a table of the normal curve, to normalized standard scores with a mean of 10 and a standard deviation of 3 for each cluster. Some smoothing was performed to adjust for sampling irregularities on all intervals studied; however, the age intervals for most combined scores exhibited adequately stable increases over the age range so that they were chosen for use.

Finally, the scores for the seven clusters were summed to create three composites, named for simplicity as Social, Speech, and Symbolic, and a total. The three composites were based on the original conceptual model for the CSBS and the results of a factor analysis of the cluster scores of the CSBS DP Behavior Sample reported in the section on Construct Validity later in this chapter. The CSBS DP composites were derived from the clusters as follows:

- Social (sum of Emotion and Eye Gaze, Communication, and Gestures)
- Speech (sum of Sounds and Words)
- Symbolic (sum of Understanding and Object Use)

The same methods described for the clusters were used to construct the norms based on normalized standard scores with a mean of 10 and a standard deviation of 3 for the composites and a mean of 100 and a standard deviation of 15 for the total.

The percentile ranks and standard scores for each of the three components are presented in the Appendixes. The seven cluster scores, three composites, and the total score may all be expressed as standard scores and percentile ranks. Teachers and parents are familiar and comfortable with percentile ranks as a method of ranking a student's performance. Salvia and Ysseldyke wrote that they, "favor the use of percentile ranks. These unpretentious scores require the fewest assumptions for accurate interpretation" (1988, p. 93). However, because percentile ranks cannot be meaningfully added, subtracted, or averaged the way that standard scores can, the standard scores are suggested for use in comparing an individual child's cluster, composite, and total scores (Hutchinson, 1996).

Score differences between males and females were studied during the analysis of the standardization data, and the results supported the construction of a single set of norms for males and females rather than separate norms by gender. The gender analyses are discussed in the section on construct validity later in this chapter.

RELIABILITY

As with any test, examiners wish to know if the results obtained from a single administration are reliable. Test reliability refers to the consistency with which the items on a test provide a stable score of the abilities being measured. Any discussion of reliability should begin with the observation that reliability as much as validity is meaningful only within the context in which the test is used. Thus, an examination of CSBS DP results must consider the conditions under which the test was administered, the similarity between the examinee and the sample with whom comparisons are to be made, and the type of decisions expected to follow from test results. In short, there are many aspects of reliability, and there are corresponding methods for estimating each. Four common methods are examined below because they help answer four common questions:

- How does performance vary from item to item?
- How is the test's measurement error reflected when reporting performance?
- How does performance on the test change over time?
- How does performance on the test vary with the rater?

Internal Consistency

Internal consistency reliability coefficients express the degree to which the parts (in the case of CSBS DP, the individual items) in an evaluation instrument measure the same characteristic. Thus, an internal consistency coefficient helps to answer the first question: How much alike are the items on the test? The more that all items in a test measure the same variable, the higher we expect the internal consistency coefficient to be. Internal consistency coefficients are useful because they provide an estimate of the reliability of a test from a single administration and because they are not affected by changes in performance due to instruction or treatment; however, because internal consistency coefficients are influenced by a test's length and by the relative difficulties of the items in the test, one cannot always conclude from a high coefficient that all of the items in the test measure the same characteristic.

Internal consistency coefficients (Cronbach's coefficient alpha) are reported by age intervals in Table 7.7 for the CSBS DP Infant-Toddler Checklist, CSBS DP Caregiver Questionnaire, and CSBS DP Behavior Sample cluster, composite, and total scores. Internal consistency was estimated using Cronbach's coefficient alpha, which is based on the average split-half correlation coefficients among all of the individual items. These coefficients treat the individual items as polychotomous and should be regarded as conservative estimates of the internal consistency of the respective scores. The raw internal reliability coefficients of the clusters, composites, and total for all three components of the CSBS DP are very high, ranging from .86 to .93, and indicate a high degree of internal consistency.

Standard Error of Measurement and Confidence Intervals

A major advantage of reliability coefficients is that they allow comparison between the reliability of different subtests or tests; however, these coefficients are not easily interpreted in terms of a particular child's score on a subtest or test. The standard error of measurement (SEM) employs the reliability coefficient to express the reliability of a subtest or test in terms of the obtained scores. That is, the SEM takes into account both the reliability of the test and the variability of performance, with the result expressed in the same unit of measurement as the obtained score. The formula used for calculating SEM is as follows:

$$\text{SEM} = \text{SD}\sqrt{(1\text{-Alpha})}$$

Thus, the SEM allows us to answer the second question: How is the test's measurement error reflected when reporting performance? Theoretically, the SEM describes a distance on either side of the child's *true score*—the score the child would receive if the test were perfectly reliable (i.e., if there were no measurement error associated with the test). However, because our only estimate of this theoretical *true score* is the child's obtained score, we use the SEM to build a range of scores around the obtained score. This range of scores around the obtained score permits us to express the child's performance in terms of an interval or band of error, rather than as a single, fixed score point with no indication of measurement error. We can also describe the degree of confidence associated with the band of error, and we can construct different confidence intervals for different levels of confidence. Of course, the larger the band of error the more confident we can be that the child's *true score* falls within the interval. To determine the bands of error, SEMs are multiplied by 1.0 for 68% confidence intervals, 1.65 for 90% confidence intervals, and 1.96 for 95% confidence intervals. Then, this number is added and subtracted from the score. For example, the 95% confidence interval is the score ±1.96 x SEM.

SEMs are presented in the Appendixes for all cluster, composite, and total scores on the norms tables and are reported in standard score units along with 68%, 90%, and 95% confidence intervals. Confidence intervals can be easily calculated using the norms tables by adding and subtracting the weighted SEM from the standard score. The examiner should apply the bands of error to standard scores for the clusters, composites, and total scores to form the desired confidence interval.

Table 7.7. Internal consistency reliability coefficients of the Infant-Toddler Checklist, Caregiver Questionnaire, and Behavior Sample

Infant-Toddler Checklist

	n	*Mean*	*SD*	*Minimum*	*Maximum*	Coefficient alpha *Raw*	Coefficient alpha *Standardized*
Clusters							
Emotion and Eye Gaze	2188	7.04	1.00	1	8	.90	.96
Communication	2188	5.75	1.80	0	8	.89	.96
Gestures	2188	6.53	2.88	0	10	.88	.96
Sounds	2188	6.27	1.54	0	8	.89	.96
Words	2188	2.44	1.88	0	6	.89	.96
Understanding	2188	4.03	1.35	0	6	.89	.96
Object Use	2188	6.79	2.75	0	11	.88	.96
Composites							
Social	2188	19.31	4.91	2	26	.87	.95
Speech	2188	8.71	3.06	0	14	.88	.95
Symbolic	2188	10.82	3.85	0	17	.87	.95
Total	**2188**	**38.84**	**10.79**	**6**	**57**	**.93**	**.95**

Caregiver Questionnaire

	n	*Mean*	*SD*	*Minimum*	*Maximum*	Coefficient alpha *Raw*	Coefficient alpha *Standardized*
Clusters							
Emotion and Eye Gaze	790	13.43	1.63	5	16	.90	.97
Communication	790	14.48	4.54	0	20	.89	.96
Gestures	790	9.66	2.82	0	12	.90	.96
Sounds	790	11.04	3.46	1	16	.90	.96
Words	790	9.61	7.57	0	24	.88	.96
Understanding	790	15.63	7.01	0	24	.88	.96
Object Use	790	15.79	7.08	0	27	.88	.96
Composites							
Social	790	37.58	7.83	9	48	.88	.96
Speech	790	20.65	10.42	1	40	.88	.96
Symbolic	790	31.42	13.49	2	51	.87	.95
Total	**790**	**89.65**	**29.14**	**13**	**139**	**.93**	**.95**

Behavior Sample

	n	*Mean*	*SD*	*Minimum*	*Maximum*	Coefficient alpha *Raw*	Coefficient alpha *Standardized*
Clusters							
Emotion and Eye Gaze	337	13.89	2.98	3	18	.89	.94
Communication	337	16.93	3.41	1	24	.88	.93
Gestures	337	13.48	4.04	0	22	.88	.94
Sounds	337	13.16	6.83	0	26	.87	.93
Words	337	7.76	8.35	0	28	.87	.93
Understanding	337	12.12	8.63	0	24	.87	.93
Object Use	337	13.13	4.99	0	24	.88	.93
Composites							
Social	337	44.31	8.46	8	62	.87	.93
Speech	337	20.93	14.34	0	54	.86	.93
Symbolic	337	25.25	12.09	0	48	.86	.93
Total	**337**	**90.49**	**29.57**	**9**	**151**	**.90**	**.92**

SD = standard deviation

Using the CSBS DP Infant-Toddler Checklist, following is an example of calculating a confidence interval for a composite score. On the Social Composite of the Infant-Toddler Checklist, a 12-month-old child's raw score = 20. The standard score for this raw score = 11 (63rd percentile) and the SEM for the Social Composite standard score = 1.1.

68% Confidence Interval = 11 ± 1.1 = 9.9 to 12.1
90% Confidence Interval = 11 ± 1.8 = 9.2 to 12.8
95% Confidence Interval = 11 ± 2.1 = 8.9 to 13.1

This calculation gives you 68% confidence that this child's true score is somewhere between 10 and 12 and 95% confidence that it is between 9 and 13.

Using the CSBS DP Behavior Sample, following is an example of calculating a confidence interval for a total score. On the Total of the Behavior Sample, a 20-month old child's raw score = 42. The standard score for this raw score = 71 (3rd percentile) and the SEM for the Total standard score = 4.8.

68% Confidence Interval = 71 ± 4.8 = 66.2 to 75.8
90% Confidence Interval = 71 ± 7.9 = 63.1 to 78.9
95% Confidence Interval = 71 ± 9.4 = 61.6 to 80.4

This calculation gives you 68% confidence that this child's true score is somewhere between 66 and 76 and 95% confidence that it is between 62 and 80.

Test–Retest Stability

An important question for examiners using test results to monitor change is the third one noted in the list: How does performance on the test change over time? The term *stability* is often used to describe the consistency of test and retest results of subjects whose relative performance has not changed. Thus, to the extent that the test yields the same results for children, we consider it to be a stable, or reliable, measure. If, however, the relative standing of the children changes over time because of development or learning, we would expect the retest to yield results different from the test. Therefore, assessing stability requires us to compare test and retest scores where development or learning has had little or no effect on the child's relative standing in the group. Test–retest reliability coefficients describe the degree of relationship between scores obtained at two different times.

The test and retest scores of children who were retested within a year of the initial administration were compared to examine the stability of the CSBS DP scores over time. For the CSBS DP Infant-Toddler Checklist, retests were available for 167 children with a mean age of 13.2 months at the initial test (SD = 3.7) and a mean age of 17.3 months at retest (SD = 3.8). For the CSBS DP Caregiver Questionnaire, retests were available for 128 children with a mean age of 13.9 months at the initial test (SD = 3.5) and a mean age of 18.1 months at retest (SD = 3.6). For the CSBS DP Behavior Sample, retests were available for 76 children with a mean age of 16.3 months at the initial test (SD = 2.5) and a mean age of 20.3 months at retest (SD = 2.4).

Table 7.8 reports a series of statistics for the children who had retests for the Infant-Toddler Checklist, Caregiver Questionnaire, and Behavior Sample for both raw and standard composite and total scores. Table 7.8 lists the means and standard deviations of the test, retest, and differences between the mean scores for the two administrations. Pearson product moment correlation coefficients (r) were calculated to examine the relationship between the test and retest scores and are reported in

Table 7.8. Test–retest reliabilities of raw and standard scores for the Infant-Toddler Checklist, Caregiver Questionnaire, and Behavior Sample

Infant-Toddler Checklist

		Test		Retest			Retest minus test				
	n	*Mean*	*SD*	*Mean*	*SD*	*MD*	*r*	*p*	*t*	*p*	*Effect size*
Raw scores											
Composites											
Social	167	17.81	5.84	20.73	4.48	2.92	.79	<.001	10.61	<.001	0.57***
Speech	167	7.72	2.95	9.62	3.01	1.90	.82	<.001	13.56	<.001	0.64**
Symbolic	167	10.00	3.96	12.68	3.46	2.68	.80	<.001	14.41	<.001	0.72**
Total	**167**	**35.53**	**11.68**	**43.04**	**9.75**	**7.50**	**.88**	**<.001**	**17.59**	**<.001**	**0.70****
Standard scores											
Composites											
Social	167	9.90	3.56	9.99	3.45	0.09	.72	<.001	0.44	ns	0.03
Speech	167	10.13	3.31	10.24	3.58	0.11	.67	<.001	0.52	ns	0.03
Symbolic	167	10.40	3.02	10.67	3.63	0.27	.65	<.001	1.22	ns	0.08
Total	**167**	**100.29**	**16.09**	**100.40**	**15.62**	**0.11**	**.86**	**<.001**	**0.17**	**ns**	**0.01**

Caregiver Questionnaire

		Test		Retest			Retest minus test				
	n	*Mean*	*SD*	*Mean*	*SD*	*MD*	*r*	*p*	*t*	*p*	*Effect size*
Raw scores											
Composites											
Social	128	33.74	9.00	38.12	7.39	4.38	.77	<.001	8.57	<.001	0.53**
Speech	128	14.55	7.63	21.18	10.23	6.63	.79	<.001	11.82	<.001	0.74**
Symbolic	128	21.90	11.83	32.02	12.12	10.12	.81	<.001	15.41	<.001	0.84***
Total	**128**	**70.19**	**25.31**	**91.31**	**26.26**	**21.12**	**.86**	**<.001**	**17.16**	**<.001**	**0.82*****
Standard scores											
Composites											
Social	128	9.24	3.11	9.47	3.25	0.23	.71	<.001	1.05	ns	0.07
Speech	128	9.37	3.13	9.20	3.09	0.17	.74	<.001	−0.86	ns	−0.05
Symbolic	128	8.64	2.67	8.80	2.59	0.16	.81	<.001	1.08	ns	0.06
Total	**128**	**94.85**	**14.43**	**95.33**	**13.95**	**0.48**	**.87**	**<.001**	**0.74**	**ns**	**0.03**

* Small effect size; ** Medium effect size; *** Large effect size; SD = standard deviation; MD = mean difference; ns = not significant

(Continued)

Table 7.8. *(Continued)*

	Behavior Sample										
		Test		Retest			Retest minus test				
	n	*Mean*	*SD*	*Mean*	*SD*	*MD*	*r*	*p*	*t*	*p*	*Effect size*
Raw scores											
Composites											
Social	76	39.99	12.84	42.14	12.22	2.15	.88	<.001	3.01	<.001	0.17
Speech	76	12.95	11.18	20.53	15.59	7.58	.89	<.001	8.65	<.001	0.57**
Symbolic	76	18.84	11.36	26.80	13.02	7.96	.76	<.001	8.11	<.001	0.65**
Total	**76**	**71.78**	**31.08**	**89.47**	**36.51**	**17.69**	**.92**	**<.001**	**10.69**	**<.001**	**0.52****
Standard scores											
Composites											
Social	76	9.39	3.75	8.99	3.76	–0.41	.77	<.001	–1.40	ns	–0.11
Speech	76	9.03	3.22	8.8	3.44	–0.22	.91	<.001	–1.36	ns	–0.07
Symbolic	76	9.12	3.32	9.03	3.70	–0.09	.79	<.001	–0.35	ns	–0.03
Total	**76**	**95.82**	**17.68**	**94.51**	**18.71**	**–1.30**	**.93**	**<.001**	**–1.67**	**ns**	**–0.07**

* Small effect size; ** Medium effect size; *** Large effect size; SD = standard deviation; MD = mean difference; ns = not significant

Table 7.8 along with the significance level of the correlations. The Pearson correlation coefficient evaluates the strength of a relationship and ranges in value from –1 to +1. This coefficient indicates the degree that low or high scores on one variable (i.e., the extent that scores fall below or above the mean) tend to go with low or high scores on another variable (Tabachnick & Fidell, 2001). Correlation coefficients of .10, .30, and .50, regardless of sign, are interpreted as small, medium, and large coefficients, respectively, in the behavioral sciences (Cohen, 1988). All raw and standard score coefficients were significant and large, ranging from .65 to .93.

Differences between the test and retest scores were analyzed by calculating a *t* test of means for paired samples. The paired-samples *t* test evaluates whether the mean difference between the test and retest scores is significantly different from zero. The results of the *t* test and the level of significance are reported in Table 7.8. These results indicate that the mean retest raw scores were significantly greater than the mean initial test raw scores for all composite and total scores for the Infant-Toddler Checklist, Caregiver Questionnaire, and Behavior Sample. In contrast, there were no significant differences between the standard scores from test to retest.

Effect sizes are also reported because they are useful for estimating the amount of growth over time and because they provide useful comparisons independent of sample size. The *d* statistic was computed as the effect size index by dividing the mean of the paired differences by the average of the standard deviations for the two samples. The average of the standard deviations was used because the variances for the two samples were not equal. When *d* equals 0, the distributions of the two samples are not different. As *d* diverges from 0, the effect size becomes larger. Regardless of sign, *d* values of .2, .5, and .8 represent small, medium, and large effect sizes, respectively (Cohen, 1988). The effect sizes for all of the raw scores are medium or large with only one exception. The exception is the Social composite for the CSBS DP Behavior Sample, which is likely limited by a ceiling effect at retest. In contrast, the effect sizes for none of the standard scores for the CSBS DP Infant-Toddler Checklist, CSBS DP Caregiver Questionnaire, and CSBS DP Behavior Sample can be classified even as small, indicating that there are not appreciable differences in standard scores from test to retest. The effect sizes are consistent with the results of the *t* tests.

Taken together, these results indicate that the CSBS DP Infant-Toddler Checklist, CSBS DP Caregiver Questionnaire, and CSBS Behavior Sample detect growth over short periods of time, based on changes in raw scores from test to retest. Furthermore, these results show that the Infant-Toddler Checklist, Caregiver Questionnaire, and Behavior Sample produce relatively stable rankings of children, even when these children show significant improvement over a short period of time, based on the strong correlations of the raw and standards scores from test to retest and the stability of the standard scores from test to retest. The test–retest data provide additional evidence of high reliability for the CSBS DP.

Inter-rater Reliability

A fourth question addressing reliability is whether a child's performance is judged similarly by different raters, when judgments are required in scoring. This is not a concern for the Infant-Toddler Checklist or Caregiver Questionnaire because parents complete each and the scores are simply tabulated. Inter-rater reliability is an important consideration for the Behavior Sample because the rater must make ongoing judgments about the occurrence or nonoccurrence of behaviors. A study of inter-rater reliability was conducted by comparing the scores of two independent raters using videotapes of Behavior Samples of 52 children, which represents 15% of the standardization sample. The two raters participated in the training for the standardization of the CSBS DP provided by the first author and scored the vast majority of the Behavior Samples used in the norms. The 52 samples were selected randomly from the full age range because the intended use of the CSBS DP is with children between 12 and 24 months with a range of abilities. Thus, although each rater scored a larger number of samples overall, the study focused on the 52 children who were scored by both raters.

Scoring the CSBS DP Behavior Sample requires judgments about behaviors in events or ongoing interaction, not performance on discrete trials or time intervals. Therefore, point-by-point agreement using Cohen's kappa is not applicable with this type of measurement system. Estimates of inter-rater reliability were obtained by calculating generalizability (*g*) or intraclass correlation coefficients between the pair of raters. The *g* coefficient is a measure of the source and magnitude of variance accounted for by the subjects and the raters and is used with similar measurement systems in the research literature (e.g., McCathren, Yoder, & Warren, 2000; McWilliam & Ware, 1994). The *g* coefficients for the cluster, composite, and total scores for the pair of raters based on 52 samples are shown in Table 7.9.

A *g* coefficient approaches 1 as the variance accounted for by the subjects is large in comparison with the variance accounted for by raters (see Bakeman & Gottman, 1997, for an explanation of generalizability theory). *G* coefficients that are in the range of .5–.7 are considered acceptable for demonstrating inter-rater reliability (Mitchel, 1979). The *g* coefficients for the pair of raters indicate that CSBS DP raters exhibit high inter-rater reliability for all clusters and very high for the composites and total. There was only one cluster on which the *g* coefficient was below .80, and this was for Gestures. The *g* coefficients for the composites and total would be considered very high, all at or above .90.

Table 7.9. Generalizability (*g*) coefficients for two examiners rating 52 Behavior Samples

	g coefficient
Clusters	
Emotion and Eye Gaze	.88
Communication	.89
Gestures	.73
Sounds	.91
Words	.92
Understanding	.95
Object Use	.89
Composites	
Social	.90
Speech	.94
Symbolic	.94
Total	**.97**

VALIDITY

The concluding section of this chapter poses a series of questions about the validity of CSBS DP scores and decisions based on those scores. In simplest terms, *validity* is the extent to which judgments based on a test are accurate and appropriate for the intended purpose (Messick, 1989). Validity is generally regarded as evidence that a test measures what it purports to measure, and various types or sources of validity are distinguished by test makers and critics. Four major aspects of validity are reported: 1) *content validity*, or logical and theoretical support for the content and organization of items; 2) *face validity*, or the extent to which the test appears to measure particular behaviors; 3) *construct validity*, or statistical evidence that the test measures the construct or constructs intended by its authors; and 4) *criterion validity*, which includes evidence of agreement between scores on the test and scores on a criterion measure already regarded as valid.

Although these distinctions provide a useful framework for organizing evidence related to an instrument's validity, they should not be thought of as different kinds of validity, nor should they be thought of as substitutes for each other. We should not attribute validity to a test; validity is an issue of test use and the application of test information to interpretation and decision-making. As Messick noted, "Validity always refers to the degree to which empirical evidence and theoretical rationales support the adequacy and appropriateness of interpretations and actions based on test scores" (1989, p. 13). Ultimately, the validity of CSBS DP use will depend on how the results are applied to decisions about children's communication and symbolic behavior.

Content Validity

Judgments of content validity rely on a clear definition of the domain tested and the design of the test in relation to the domain, or what Messick called "the relevance and representativeness of the test items with respect to the domain" (1989, p. 17). The more clearly specified the rationale for the content, the more easily one can begin to assess the test's content validity. Evidence that the CSBS DP targets relevant domains of communication and symbolic behavior is provided in Chapter 2, which cites a rationale and relevant research literature that supports the instrument. The communication and symbolic behaviors measured are well documented in the literature as important skills that develop over the first 2 years of life. Statistical evidence supporting a developmental progression of behaviors measured is provided under the discussion of construct validity. All three components—the Infant-Toddler Checklist, the Caregiver Questionnaire, and the Behavior Sample—were designed to evaluate the same seven cluster areas derived from the research literature on prelinguistic predictors, reviewed in Chapter 2. Statistical evidence supporting the relationship among the three components is provided under the discussion of criterion validity.

Face Validity

Face validity is the appearance of validity. That is, face validity is judged by appearance rather than by a detailed analysis of content as is done to establish content validity. For this reason, face validity has often been judged harshly and is often ignored. Researchers use the term *ecological validity* to describe the degree to which the setting of an experiment is similar to the setting to which the results are to be generalized. Recent proponents of *authentic assessment* argue that the ecological validity of an evaluation/assessment is related to how the participants (e.g., a student and the teacher or parent and clinician) judge the appearance of a test. In these cases, at least, face validity may have to be considered an important aspect of an evaluation/assessment because the student and teacher or parent and clinician may show little commitment to the evaluation/assessment if they view its context and form as inauthentic or irrelevant.

For similar reasons, the CSBS DP procedures attempt to ensure the ecological validity of the information obtained by maximizing the role of the caregiver and using a naturalistic context. Bronfenbrenner has cautioned that our understanding of child development has been based on "the strange behavior of children in strange situations with strange adults for the briefest possible periods of time" (1979, p. viii). In the CSBS DP, the role of a caregiver as informant and participant and the use of sampling procedures with common toys and typical play activities are features that contribute to a more naturalistic context. This is usually not found with most tests made up of subtests with contrived tasks and independent items ordered by difficulty.

Construct Validity

Construct validity is statistical evidence that the test measures the construct or constructs it purports to measure. The statistical evidence can take the form of interpretable quantitative relationships between the test scores and other variables known to be related to the construct. Construct validity can also be shown through a study of the relationships among the various components of the test. In either case, the relationships of interest are those that could be predicted from the various elements in the test makers' theory or model of performance. Four types of construct validity data are presented in this section: developmental progression of scores, intercorrelations, gender differences, and principal components analysis.

Developmental Progression of Scores

A test that measures communication and symbolic behaviors from 6 to 24 months of age should demonstrate growth and age differentiation because these skills show rapid development during the first 2 years of life. Tables 7.10, 7.11, and 7.12 report raw scores by age intervals (of 1–4 months) for the Infant-Toddler Checklist, Caregiver Questionnaire, and Behavior Sample. The pattern of score increases on nearly all of the cluster, composite, and total scores are consistent with growth on these aspects of communication and symbolic behaviors during this period of early development. Table 7.10 reports the means and standard deviations of the raw scores for the Infant-Toddler Checklist composites and total by 1-month age intervals. The means and standard deviations of the weighted raw scores for the clusters, composites, and total are reported in Table 7.11 for the Caregiver Questionnaire and Table 7.12 for the Behavior Sample for the age intervals represented in the norms tables.

Table 7.10. Means and standard deviations (SD) of composite and total raw scores for the Infant-Toddler Checklist, by age in months

		Composite						Total	
		Social		Speech		Symbolic			
Age (months)	*n*	*Mean*	*SD*	*Mean*	*SD*	*Mean*	*SD*	*Mean*	*SD*
6	50	10.00	2.95	3.74	1.76	4.32	1.48	18.06	4.70
7	42	11.31	2.98	4.17	1.96	4.71	1.78	20.19	5.33
8	77	13.12	4.62	5.48	2.24	5.69	1.82	24.29	7.31
9	126	13.06	3.88	5.59	2.05	6.09	1.92	24.74	6.38
10	86	16.02	3.82	6.99	1.91	7.30	2.09	30.31	6.29
11	312	18.24	4.21	7.68	2.19	9.13	2.74	35.05	7.70
12	296	19.06	3.96	7.81	2.18	9.58	2.62	36.46	7.41
13	121	19.43	4.36	8.36	2.09	10.44	2.63	38.23	7.70
14	128	20.62	3.52	8.77	2.14	11.41	2.63	40.80	6.76
15	174	21.13	3.26	9.19	2.11	12.03	2.29	42.36	6.28
16	98	21.77	3.62	9.87	2.30	13.22	2.60	44.86	7.40
17	99	22.35	2.66	10.35	2.21	13.62	2.13	46.32	5.65
18	133	21.72	3.60	10.59	2.74	13.77	2.37	46.08	7.77
19	107	22.50	2.93	10.93	2.74	13.79	2.74	47.22	7.06
20	84	22.30	3.04	11.26	2.72	14.12	2.38	47.68	6.72
21	87	22.84	2.79	11.60	2.49	14.89	1.90	49.32	5.60
22	82	22.23	3.45	11.84	2.18	14.96	2.47	49.04	7.08
23	50	22.20	3.04	11.80	2.77	14.50	2.56	48.50	7.12
24	36	22.39	3.02	11.94	2.12	15.03	1.99	49.36	5.60
Total	**2188**								

The developmental trends portrayed in Tables 7.10–7.12 indicate that substantial growth is measured by the Infant-Toddler Checklist, Caregiver Questionnaire, and Behavior Sample across the age span in the standardization sample. The composite raw scores increase at different rates across the age span represented in the standardization sample for the Infant-Toddler Checklist, Caregiver Questionnaire, and Behavior Sample. The mean for the Social composite is higher then either the Speech or Symbolic Composites at the younger age groups. Furthermore, the largest change on the Social Composite is evident under 12 months for the Infant-Toddler Checklist and Caregiver Questionnaire, while that for the Speech and Symbolic Composites is evident over 12 months of age. The pattern of developmental growth in Tables 7.10–7.12 indicates that the Social Composite and the clusters that comprise it measure skills that typically develop between 6 and 18 months of age and the Speech and Symbolic Composites and corresponding clusters measure skills that continue to develop through 24 months of age.

Intercorrelations

An important issue in the use of the CSBS DP is the degree to which the individual items provide different information about the child's development. This issue was previously addressed under the topic of internal consistency with data in Table 7.7. Another approach to examining this issue is to study the intercorrelations among various subtests of a test, in this case the CSBS DP item composites and clusters. Traditionally, this approach is considered with construct validity. Tables 7.13–7.15 present a raw score intercorrelation matrix of *composite* scores for the Infant-Toddler Checklist, Caregiver Questionnaire, and Behavior Sample, respectively, for 6-month age intervals and the

Table 7.11. Means and standard deviations (SD) of cluster, composite, and total weighted raw scores for the Caregiver Questionnaire, by age in months

		Clusters							
		Emotion		Communication		Gestures		Sounds	
Age (months)	*n*	*Mean*	*SD*	*Mean*	*SD*	*Mean*	*SD*	*Mean*	*SD*
6–7	12	13.17	0.83	5.08	3.48	2.25	2.01	6.00	3.02
8–9	47	12.62	1.94	6.70	4.34	4.26	2.44	7.28	3.20
10–11	53	13.42	1.46	10.47	3.25	6.81	2.62	9.02	2.61
12	71	13.14	1.62	12.93	4.43	8.76	2.33	9.42	2.90
13–14	107	13.48	1.74	14.16	4.02	9.52	2.45	10.21	2.78
15–16	129	13.60	1.65	15.49	3.54	10.42	1.98	11.20	2.92
17–18	114	13.56	1.63	15.68	3.35	10.66	1.53	11.77	3.10
19–20	113	13.52	1.64	16.50	3.20	11.04	1.61	12.74	3.23
21–22	89	13.54	1.52	16.81	2.69	11.17	1.24	12.78	3.08
23–24	55	13.47	1.41	16.91	2.86	11.02	1.82	12.85	3.45

		Clusters					
		Words		Understanding		Object use	
Age (months)	*n*	*Mean*	*SD*	*Mean*	*SD*	*Mean*	*SD*
6–7	12	0.08	0.29	3.42	2.31	3.25	1.36
8–9	47	1.55	3.38	5.23	3.63	4.60	2.36
10–11	53	2.00	3.08	7.53	3.92	6.64	3.20
12	71	3.97	3.74	10.55	5.23	10.89	4.21
13–14	107	6.21	4.45	13.35	5.48	13.66	4.91
15–16	129	8.95	5.53	16.28	5.09	16.49	5.16
17–18	114	10.98	6.20	18.45	4.99	17.96	4.83
19–20	113	15.29	6.81	20.16	5.15	20.93	5.05
21–22	89	15.62	6.95	20.49	4.82	21.46	4.45
23–24	55	17.04	6.89	21.44	4.50	21.55	5.52

		Composites							
		Social		Speech		Symbolic		**Total**	
Age (months)	*n*	*Mean*	*SD*	*Mean*	*SD*	*Mean*	*SD*	*Mean*	*SD*
6–7	12	20.50	5.47	6.08	2.97	6.67	3.11	33.25	9.03
8–9	47	23.57	7.59	8.83	5.55	9.83	5.35	42.23	16.65
10–11	53	30.70	5.77	11.02	4.71	14.17	6.49	55.89	14.03
12	71	34.83	7.24	13.39	5.91	21.44	8.54	69.66	18.39
13–14	107	37.16	6.95	16.43	6.40	27.01	9.50	80.60	19.94
15–16	129	39.51	6.14	20.16	7.76	32.77	9.33	92.43	20.03
17–18	114	39.89	5.37	22.75	8.51	36.41	8.91	99.06	19.28
19–20	113	41.06	5.62	28.04	9.57	41.09	9.43	110.19	21.73
21–22	89	41.52	4.33	28.39	9.63	41.96	8.02	111.87	18.98
23–24	55	41.40	4.75	29.89	10.04	42.98	9.20	114.27	21.40
Total	**790**								

entire sample. These correlations suggest that somewhat different skills or abilities are measured by each composite, although the different composites tend to demonstrate similar distributions of scores. The Speech and Symbolic Composites are generally more strongly related to each other than either one is to the Social Composite.

These patterns are further supported by the intercorrelations among cluster scores. Tables 7.16–7.18 present a raw score intercorrelation matrix of *cluster* scores for the Infant-Toddler Checklist, Caregiver Questionnaire, and Behavior Sample, respectively. Inspection of these tables reveals a pattern of moderate correlations among most cluster scores when all ages are combined. When the 6-month age intervals are examined,

Table 7.12. Means and standard deviations of cluster, composite, and total weighted raw scores for the Behavior Sample, by age in months

		Clusters							
		Emotion		Communication		Gesture		Sounds	
Age (months)	*n*	*Mean*	*SD*	*Mean*	*SD*	*Mean*	*SD*	*Mean*	*SD*
12–14	82	12.95	3.65	15.41	4.12	12.23	3.96	8.65	5.53
15–17	76	13.84	2.76	16.26	2.94	13.00	3.59	11.59	5.62
18–20	76	14.13	3.02	17.37	3.20	13.78	4.18	14.36	6.27
21–24	103	14.50	2.29	18.32	2.58	14.62	4.03	17.04	6.55

		Clusters					
		Words		Understanding		Objects	
Age (months)	*n*	*Mean*	*SD*	*Mean*	*SD*	*Mean*	*SD*
12–14	82	1.52	6.28	5.52	2.48	8.39	3.45
15–17	76	4.68	7.90	9.71	4.95	12.11	3.70
18–20	76	8.91	7.92	13.97	7.92	14.78	4.80
21–24	103	14.16	6.88	17.80	8.96	16.44	3.71

		Composites							
		Social		Speech		Symbolic		**Total**	
Age (months)	*n*	*Mean*	*SD*	*Mean*	*SD*	*Mean*	*SD*	*Mean*	*SD*
12–14	82	40.60	10.04	10.17	7.26	13.91	8.03	64.68	20.87
15–17	76	43.11	7.11	16.28	9.82	21.82	9.67	81.20	20.70
18–20	76	45.28	8.31	23.26	13.29	28.75	11.06	97.29	27.47
21–24	103	47.45	6.70	31.19	14.67	34.23	8.32	112.87	22.89
Total	**337**								

Table 7.13. Intercorrelations among composite raw scores of the Infant-Toddler Checklist for children in the standardized sample, by age

	n	Social	Speech
Ages 6–11 months			
Composites	693		
Speech		.65	
Symbolic		.69	.65
Ages 12–17 months			
Composites	916		
Speech		.54	
Symbolic		.62	.63
Ages 18–24 months			
Composites	579		
Speech		.51	
Symbolic		.57	.65
Ages 6–24 months			
Composites	2188		
Speech		.70	
Symbolic		.76	.78

p<.001 unless otherwise noted
*p<.01
**p<.05
ns = not significant

Table 7.14. Intercorrelations among composite raw scores of the Caregiver Questionnaire for the children in the standardization sample, by age

	n	Social	Speech
Age 6–11 months			
Composites	112		
Speech		.59	
Symbolic		.73	.64
Age 12–17 months			
Composites	359		
Speech		.54	
Symbolic		.73	.68
Age 18–24 months			
Composites	319		
Speech		.45	
Symbolic		.73	.67
Age 6–24 months			
Composites	790		
Speech		.63	
Symbolic		.81	.79

$p<.001$ unless otherwise noted
*$p<.01$
**$p<.05$
ns = not significant

stronger correlations are generally found among clusters within the same composites and weaker correlations are found among clusters that are from different composites.

Gender Differences

The pattern of score increases by age may be contrasted with the pattern of score differences by gender. Whereas substantial changes in communication and symbolic behaviors may be predicted with increasing age during this period of early development, substantial differences between females and males would not be as predictable at these early ages. For this reason, a group of males and females were matched on age (to the tenth of a month) and race. Table 7.19 presents the comparison of the scores of the two matched groups on the Infant-Toddler Checklist, Caregiver Questionnaire, and Behavior Sample

Table 7.15. Intercorrelations among composite raw scores of the Behavior Sample for children in the standardized sample, by age

	n	Social	Speech
Age 12–17 months			
Composites	158		
Social		.47	
Symbolic		.48	.59
Age 18–24 months			
Composites	179		
Speech		.52	
Symbolic		.53	.48
Age 12–24 months			
Composites	337		
Speech		.48	
Symbolic		.53	.65

$p<.001$ unless otherwise noted
*$p<.01$
**$p<.05$
ns = not significant

Table 7.16. Intercorrelations among cluster raw scores of the Infant-Toddler Checklist for children in the standardization sample, by age

Clusters	Emotion	Communication	Gestures	Sounds	Words	Understanding
Age 6–11 months						
n = 693						
Communication	.54					
Gestures	.44	.58				
Sounds	.37	.45	.51			
Words	.28	.38	.60	.45		
Understanding	.44	.48	.61	.45	.58	
Object Use	.34	.42	.65	.45	.59	.62
Age 12–17 months						
n = 916						
Communication	.55					
Gestures	.42	.54				
Sounds	.38	.41	.42			
Words	.26	.32	.45	.49		
Understanding	.43	.42	.52	.44	.60	
Object Use	.39	.41	.53	.41	.50	.56
Age 18–24 months						
n = 579						
Communication	.50					
Gestures	.46	.53				
Sounds	.34	.40	.47			
Words	.27	.36	.42	.65		
Understanding	.41	.40	.44	.54	.59	
Object Use	.34	.42	.46	.49	.51	.52
Age 6–24 months						
n = 2188						
Communication	.57					
Gestures	.47	.66				
Sounds	.41	.52	.59			
Words	.32	.49	.65	.60		
Understanding	.46	.57	.69	.58	.73	
Object Use	.40	.56	.73	.57	.72	.74

$p<.001$ unless otherwise noted
*$p<.01$
**$p<.05$
ns = not significant

with the result that no substantial differences were found on almost all of the clusters. Table 7.19 lists the means and standard deviations of females and males, the differences between the mean scores for the two groups, the results of a *t* test for paired samples, and the effect size of each difference. This statistical analysis is similar to that on test–retest stability reported previously in the chapter in the section on reliability.

For the CSBS DP Infant-Toddler Checklist, CSBS DP Caregiver Questionnaire, and CSBS DP Behavior Sample, the *t* tests of differences were significant at the .05 level for only one composite score, the Speech Composite for the Caregiver Questionnaire. This presumably reflects the significant difference found for the Sounds Cluster at the .05 level for the Caregiver Questionnaire. The Gesture Cluster for the Infant-Toddler Checklist also reached the .05 level-of-significance; however, norms are presented only for composite scores for the Infant-Toddler Checklist, and the Communication Composite was not significantly different for females and males. Using Cohen's (1988) classification described earlier in this chapter, only one of the effect sizes for the Behavior Sample and all but one of the effect sizes for the Caregiver Questionnaire were large enough to be considered small. Even so, none of the cluster, composite, or total scores for the Infant-Toddler Checklist, Caregiver Questionnaire, or Behavior Sample had effect sizes that would be considered

Table 7.17. Intercorrelations among cluster raw scores of the Caregiver Questionnaire for children in the standardization sample, by age

Clusters	Emotion	Communication	Gestures	Sounds	Words	Understanding
Age 6–11 months						
n = 112						
Communication	.51					
Gestures	.32	.72				
Sounds	.31	.55	.47			
Words	.08ns	.39	.50	.40		
Understanding	.33	.67	.71	.49	.60	
Object Use	.22**	.57	.60	.44	.38	.67
Age 12–17 months						
n = 359						
Communication	.51					
Gestures	.47	.65				
Sounds	.35	.41	.44			
Words	.24	.48	.47	.63		
Understanding	.42	.64	.60	.45	.65	
Object Use	.41	.63	.59	.48	.62	.73
Age 18–24 months						
n = 319						
Communication	.46					
Gestures	.37	.62				
Sounds	.30	.48	.46			
Words	.17**	.38	.38	.79		
Understanding	.40	.59	.54	.61	.60	
Object Use	.39	.62	.61	.58	.53	.62
Age 6–24 months						
n = 790						
Communication	.45					
Gestures	.36	.79				
Sounds	.33	.58	.57			
Words	.20	.58	.59	.75		
Understanding	.36	.75	.74	.64	.77	
Object Use	.33	.75	.75	.64	.74	.83

p<.001 unless otherwise noted
*p<.01
**p<.05
ns = not significant

medium or large. These data lend support to the use of one set of norms for both males and females; however, it is noteworthy that all of the differences were in the direction of females scoring higher, although the differences were negligible or small.

Principal Components Analysis

The relationship among the 20 scales of the Behavior Sample was analyzed using a principal components analysis to determine whether the scales were more interpretable by grouping them based on the obtained component solution. An analysis of the observed correlation matrix of the weighted raw scores of the CSBS DP Behavior Sample scales was conducted using a principal component analysis extraction method (Tabachnick & Fidell, 2001). Six factors had initial Eigenvalues above 1, but the number of factors to rotate was determined to be 3, based on the scree plot. Three components were rotated using a Varimax rotation method. The rotated solution is presented in Table 7.20.

The first principal component accounted for 24% of the variance. Component 1 is interpreted as a Speech Composite, with Scales 10–15, which comprise the Sounds and Words Clusters, loading very high on this factor. The second principal component

Table 7.18. Intercorrelations among cluster raw scores of the Behavior Sample for children in the standardization sample, by age

Clusters	Emotion	Communication	Gestures	Sounds	Words	Understanding
Age 12–17 months						
n = 158						
Communication	.47					
Gestures	.43	.65				
Sounds	.26	.47	.40			
Words	.19**	.29	.31	.67		
Understanding	.25*	.31	.28	.37	.57	
Object Use	.35	.46	.34	.37	.38	.39
Age 18–24 months						
n =179						
Communication	.37					
Gestures	.33	.49				
Sounds	.17**	.29	.29			
Words	.25	.28	.28	.77		
Understanding	.38	.32	.32	.49	.49	
Object Use	.42	.27	.27	.35	.35	.37
Age 12–24 months						
n = 337						
Communication	.45					
Gestures	.45	.59				
Sounds	.26	.53	.39			
Words	.26	.42	.35	.78		
Understanding	.35	.42	.35	.50	.62	
Object Use	.40	.47	.35	.47	.53	.54

p<.001 unless otherwise noted
*p<.01
**p<.05
ns = not significant

accounted for 16% of the variance. Component 2 is interpreted as a Social Composite, with Scales 1–9, which comprise the Emotion and Eye Gaze, Communication, and Gestures Clusters, loading highest on this factor. The third principal component accounted for 14% of the variance. Component 3 is interpreted as a Symbolic Composite, with Scales 16–20, which comprise the Understanding and Object Use Clusters loading highest on this factor.

It should be noted that 2 of the 20 scales loaded on two factors, Scales 3 and 16. Scale 3, Gaze/Point Following, loaded on both the Social and the Symbolic Composites. This is logical since this is a measure of both social referencing and nonverbal comprehension. Scale 16, Language Comprehension, loaded on both Speech and Symbolic Components. This is logical since this measure is strongly related to both expressive language and play. It was decided to leave the Understanding Cluster in the Symbolic Composite because children with language problems often show receptive language more closely related to play levels than expressive language levels.

Thus, the three-component solution of the principal component analysis for the Behavior Sample supported the seven clusters as well as three composites. A principal component analysis was not conducted for the Caregiver Questionnaire or the Infant-Toddler Checklist because of the very limited response scales (i.e., not yet, sometimes, often) for most of the items of these components.

Criterion Validity

Because there are so few measures designed specifically to assess the communicative and symbolic behavior of children younger than 24 months of age, criterion validity

Table 7.19. Comparisons of raw scores for the Infant-Toddler Checklist, Caregiver Questionnaire, and Behavior Sample for matched pairs of females and males in the standardized sample

Infant-Toddler Checklist

n = 253 pairs	Female		Male		Female minus male			
	Mean	*SD*	*Mean*	*SD*	*MD*	*t*	*p*	*Effect size*
Clusters								
Emotion and Eye Gaze	7.05	1.00	6.92	0.96	0.13	1.50	ns	0.13
Communication	5.64	1.89	5.64	1.77	0.00	–0.02	ns	0.00
Gestures	6.60	3.11	6.03	2.99	0.57	2.08	<.05	0.19
Sounds	6.60	1.56	6.09	1.63	0.21	1.48	ns	0.13
Words	2.56	2.04	2.32	1.93	0.24	1.37	ns	0.12
Understanding	4.04	1.42	3.87	1.39	0.17	1.36	ns	0.12
Object Use	6.91	3.07	6.56	2.63	0.35	1.37	ns	0.12
Composites								
Social	19.28	5.24	18.59	4.98	0.69	1.52	ns	0.14
Speech	8.86	3.33	8.41	3.22	0.45	1.55	ns	0.14
Symbolic	10.94	4.25	10.42	3.76	0.52	1.45	ns	0.13
Total	**39.08**	**11.85**	**37.42**	**10.96**	**1.66**	**1.64**	**ns**	**0.15**

Caregiver Questionnaire

n = 84 pairs	Female		Male		Female minus male			
	Mean	*SD*	*Mean*	*SD*	*MD*	*t*	*p*	*Effect size*
Clusters								
Emotion and Eye Gaze	13.73	1.20	13.34	1.72	0.39	1.49	ns	0.26*
Communication	15.48	4.21	14.63	4.30	0.86	1.14	ns	0.20*
Gestures	10.20	2.46	9.31	3.20	0.89	1.76	ns	0.31*
Sounds	11.55	3.00	10.16	3.44	1.39	2.44	<.05	0.43*
Words	10.30	7.59	8.02	6.94	2.28	1.78	ns	0.31*
Understanding	15.92	7.01	14.84	6.76	1.08	0.89	ns	0.16
Object Use	16.42	7.28	14.41	6.40	2.02	1.66	ns	0.29*
Composites								
Social	39.42	6.66	37.28	7.91	2.14	1.66	ns	0.29*
Speech	21.84	9.99	18.17	9.65	3.67	2.12	<.05	0.37*
Symbolic	32.34	13.89	29.25	12.59	3.09	1.32	ns	0.23*
Total	**93.61**	**28.17**	**84.70**	**27.22**	**8.91**	**1.82**	**ns**	**0.32***

Behavior Sample

n = 45 pairs	Female		Male		Female minus male			
	Mean	*SD*	*Mean*	*SD*	*MD*	*t*	*p*	*Effect size*
Clusters								
Emotion and Eye Gaze	13.89	3.51	13.44	2.99	0.44	0.65	ns	0.14
Communication	17.09	3.26	16.91	3.46	0.18	0.25	ns	0.05
Gestures	13.40	4.46	12.69	4.37	0.71	0.76	ns	0.16
Sounds	14.02	6.3	13.09	7.01	0.93	0.65	ns	0.14
Words	9.80	8.82	7.56	8.76	2.24	1.21	ns	0.26*
Understanding	11.60	8.83	11.20	9.73	0.40	0.20	ns	0.04
Object Use	13.40	5.62	12.56	4.77	0.84	0.77	ns	0.16
Composites								
Social	44.38	9.09	43.04	9.18	1.33	0.69	ns	0.15
Speech	23.82	14.43	20.64	14.77	3.18	1.03	ns	0.22*
Symbolic	25.00	13.39	23.76	12.43	1.24	0.46	ns	0.10
Total	**93.20**	**31.82**	**87.44**	**29.88**	**5.76**	**0.88**	**ns**	**0.19**

*small effect size; ** medium effect size; *** large effect size; SD = standard deviation; MD = mean difference

Table 7.20. Rotated component matrix for the Behavior Sample scales

Scales	Speech Component 1	Social Component 2	Symbolic Component 3
Emotion and Eye Gaze			
1. Gaze shifts	0.05	0.28	0.08
2. Shared positive affect	0.07	0.41	0.12
3. Gaze/point following	0.17	0.39	0.43
Communication			
4. Rate of communicating	0.15	0.74	0.21
5. Behavior regulation	0.13	0.65	0.16
6. Social interaction	0.01	0.27	0.30
7. Joint attention	0.41	0.61	0.08
Gestures			
8. Inventory of conventional gestures	0.25	0.62	0.20
9. Distal gestures	0.08	0.73	0.02
Sounds			
10. Syllables with consonants	0.79	0.45	0.13
11. Inventory of consonants	0.78	0.31	0.18
Words			
12. Words	0.88	0.25	0.34
13. Inventory of words	0.88	0.15	0.29
14. Word combinations	0.87	–0.01	0.10
15. Inventory of word combinations	0.88	–0.05	0.13
Understanding			
16. Language comprehension	0.54	0.22	0.46
Object Use			
17. Inventory of action schemes	0.17	0.22	0.82
18. Action schemes toward others	0.10	0.23	0.73
19. Sequences action schemes	0.28	0.06	0.64
20. Stacks tower of blocks	0.35	0.17	0.58
Percent of total variance	**23.94**	**16.33**	**14.20**

studies of the CSBS DP are necessarily limited; however, a series of studies were conducted to examine both concurrent and predictive validity, which are aspects of criterion validity using standardized measures of language and related abilities. Concurrent validity is evidence that scores on an instrument accurately indicate how subjects would be classified by an independent criterion administered at the same point in time, whereas predictive validity is evidence that scores on an instrument accurately predict how subjects would be classified by an independent criterion administered at a time in the future. For the CSBS DP, both concurrent and predictive validity address practical questions because they relate to how useful the scores may be in identifying children at risk for potential delays or disorders.

Concurrent Validity

The concurrent validity of the CSBS DP was evaluated by comparing standard scores among the three components—the Infant-Toddler Checklist, Caregiver Questionnaire, and Behavior Sample. Subjects were drawn from children in the standardization sample and a pool of about 50 children with communication and language delays. Since the CSBS DP will be used with children who have developmental delays, we felt that it was important to include them in the studies of concurrent validity. Children were selected for this study if they had completed two of the components at the same age (plus or minus 3 months). The relationship among the Infant-Toddler Checklist, Caregiver Questionnaire, and Behavior Sample was examined by calculating Pearson correlation coefficients on pairs of standard scores obtained from the same children. The correlation coefficients for the composite and total standard scores on the Infant-Toddler Checklist and Caregiver Questionnaire, Caregiver Questionnaire and Behavior Sample, and the Infant-Toddler Checklist and Behavior Sample are presented in Table 7.21.

Large, significant correlations were observed among all of the total scores and moderate or large, significant correlations were observed among all of the composites. Patterns of the correlations are noteworthy. The strongest correlations were observed between the Infant-Toddler Checklist and the Caregiver Questionnaire, which are both parent report measures. Very similar correlations were found between the Caregiver Questionnaire and the Behavior Sample and between the Infant-Toddler Checklist and the Behavior Sample. In comparing across composites, the strongest correlations were generally observed for the Speech Composite, followed by the Symbolic Composite. The strongest correlations were also generally observed for the oldest age group (18–24 months).

These findings support the validity of these parent report tools as a measure of early communication and symbolic abilities. The Infant-Toddler Checklist, which is a brief parent report tool, had a very strong correlation with the Caregiver Questionnaire, a more in-depth parent report tool. Furthermore, there was a strong relationship between children's standard scores on the parent report tools (i.e., Infant-Toddler Checklist and Caregiver Questionnaire) and those based on the face-to-face evaluation of the child (i.e., Behavior Sample).

Predictive Validity

The predictive validity of the CSBS DP was evaluated by comparing standard scores from the three components—the Infant-Toddler Checklist, Caregiver Questionnaire, and Behavior Sample, with children's outcomes on standardized testing at 2 and 3

Table 7.21. Correlations and total standard scores for the Infant-Toddler Checklist (ITC), Caregiver Questionnaire (CQ), and Behavior Sample (BS) administered within 3 months, by age

	n	ITC & CQ	*n*	CQ & BS	*n*	ITC & BS
Age 6–11 months						
Composites	77					
Social		.50				
Speech		.54				
Symbolic		.53				
Total		**.56**				
Age 12–17 months						
Composites	215		123		100	
Social		.77		.44		.47
Speech		.74		.63		.54
Symbolic		.71		.62		.53
Total		**.80**		**.66**		**.62**
Age 18–24 months						
Composites	202		140		84	
Social		.73		.44		.38
Speech		.84		.76		.74
Symbolic		.79		.58		.57
Total		**.88**		**.71**		**.68**

$p < .001$ unless otherwise noted
*$p < .01$
**$p < .05$
ns = not significant

years of age. The Mullen Scales of Early Learning (Mullen, 1995), which measures gross motor, fine motor, visual recognition, receptive language, and expressive language and provides an Early Learning Composite of the four cognitive scales (i.e., excluding gross motor), was used for the follow-up standardized testing. This measure was selected because it has good psychometric features, provides a cognitive composite, and also provides separate scores for receptive and expressive language. Subjects were drawn from children in the standardization sample and a pool of about 60 children at-risk for communication and language delays. Children at risk were defined as those who performed in the bottom 10th percentile based on the CSBS DP. These children were recruited from health care and child care agencies who administered the Infant-Toddler Checklist, and their families were invited to complete the Caregiver Questionnaire and Behavior Sample. About 120 typical children were randomly selected from the standardization sample in the Tallahassee region based on scores above the 10th percentile on the CSBS DP. All of these families were invited to bring their child in for follow-up standardized testing just after their second birthday and again after their third birthday.

The relationship between each of the CSBS DP components and the Mullen Scales was examined by calculating Pearson correlation coefficients on pairs of standard scores obtained from the same children. The Receptive Language Scale, Expressive Language Scale, and Learning Composite of the Mullen Scales and the Social, Speech, and Symbolic Composites and the Total of each measure of the CSBS DP were used for this analysis. The mean and standard deviation of the test scores and the children's age at administration and the correlation coefficients (r) between components are presented in Table 7.22 for the 2-year-old follow-up testing and Table 7.23 for the 3-year-old follow-up testing.

Moderate to large, significant correlations were observed among all of the scores both at 2- and 3-year-old follow-up testing. Patterns of the correlations are noteworthy. The strongest correlations were observed between the Mullen Scales and the CSBS DP Behavior Sample; both of these evaluations are face-to-face. Very similar correlations were found between the Mullen Scales and the CSBS DP Infant-Toddler Checklist and CSBS DP Caregiver Questionnaire. In comparing across composites, the strongest correlations were generally observed between the CSBS DP Speech Composite and the Expressive Language Scale of the Mullen Scales and between the CSBS DP Symbolic Composite and the Receptive Language Scale of the Mullen Scales. The strongest correlations were generally observed between the Learning Composite of the Mullen Scales and the Total of the CSBS DP. The correlations were larger at the 2-year-old follow-up testing than at the 3-year-old follow-up testing, but the relationships continued to be strong at the 3-year-old follow-up testing.

Using the same data, predictive validity was also evaluated by comparing the classifications of the child's performance based on the CSBS DP with the classification of performance based on the follow-up standardized testing at 2 and 3 years of age. First, we had to decide our criteria for being at risk on the CSBS DP and failing the follow-up testing. Many tests and state eligibility criteria use the criteria of either 2 or 1.5 standard deviations below the mean as a cutoff, which corresponds with the 2nd and 7th percentiles, respectively. However, we chose 1.25 standard deviations below the mean, which corresponds with the 10th percentile, because 10%–15% of school-age children have developmental disabilities that require special education,

Table 7.22. Correlations of standard scores for the Infant-Toddler Checklist, Caregiver Questionnaire, and Behavior Sample with the Mullen Scales of Early Learning administered at 2 years

			Mullen Scales of Early Learning										
n = 192			Receptive language			Expressive language			Leaning composite			Age (months)	
	Mean	*SD*	*Mean*	*SD*	*r*	*Mean*	*SD*	*r*	*Mean*	*SD*	*r*	*Mean*	*SD*
Infant-Toddler Checklist													
Composites			50.9	15.0		46.5	15.1		99.6	24.2		25.2	1.7
Social	9.1	3.3			.48			.43			.48		
Speech	8.5	3.1			.39			.50			.43		
Symbolic	9.4	3.2			.54			.41			.58		
Total	93.4	15.9			.54			.51			.57		
Age (months)	14.0	4.2											
n = 141													
Caregiver Questionnaire													
Composites			49.2	15.7		44.2	14.2		96.2	24.6		25.1	1.7
Social	9.4	3.3			.49			.44			.46		
Speech	8.5	2.8			.42			.52			.48		
Symbolic	8.7	2.6			.53			.53			.57		
Total	91.61	13.4			.55			.63			.59		
Age (months)	16.7	4.8											
n = 141													
Behavior Sample													
Composites			50.5	16.0		47.2	15.8		99.3	25.6		25.1	1.8
Social	9.7	3.6			.64			.50			.58		
Speech	8.8	2.9			.61			.73			.64		
Symbolic	9.8	3.5			.75			.62			.64		
Total	94.4	16.8			.74			.73			.71		
Age (months)	20.8	2.2											

Note: Mullen Scales scores for the Receptive and Expressive Language Scales are T scores (M = 50, SD = 10) and for the Learning Composite are standard scores (M = 100, SD = 15). CSBS DP scores are standard scores for the composites (M = 10, SD = 3) and Total (M = 100, SD = 15).

p < .001 unless otherwise noted
* p < .01
** p < .05
ns = not significant
SD = standard deviation

Table 7.23. Correlations of standard scores for the Infant-Toddler Checklist, Caregiver Questionnaire, and Behavior Sample with the Mullen Scales of Early Learning administered at 3 years

			Mullen Scales of Early Learning										
			Receptive language			Expressive language			Leaning composite			Age (months)	
n = 92	*Mean*	*SD*	*Mean*	*SD*	*r*	*Mean*	*SD*	*r*	*Mean*	*SD*	*r*	*Mean*	*SD*
Infant-Toddler Checklist													
Composites			49.6	12.1		52.0	13.1		106.3	24.4		37.9	2.2
Social	8.5	3.3			.33			.38			.40		
Speech	8.2	3.3			.28*			.39			.35		
Symbolic	9.0	3.3			.49			.56			.56		
Total	90.5	16.4			.40			.49			.48		
Age (months)	16.1	4.0											
n = 91													
Caregiver Questionnaire													
Composites			49.7	12.2		52.5	12.9		106.8	24.2		38.0	2.1
Social	9.4	2.9			.33*			.43			.40		
Speech	9.1	2.8			.33*			.48			.44		
Symbolic	8.9	2.4			.49								
Total	92.6	12.7			.47			.59			.57		
Age (months)	16.9	4.1											
n = 90													
Behavior Sample													
Composites			49.6	12.2		52.2	13.1		105.8	24.4		38.0	2.1
Social	10.2	3.1			.53			.60			.59		
Speech	9.6	3.2			.45			.65			.61		
Symbolic	9.2	3.4			.62			.64			.68		
Total	96.6	17.5			.59			.72			.71		
Age (months) 19.6	3.4												

Note: Mullen Scales scores for the Receptive and Expressive Language Scales are T scores (M = 50, SD = 10) and for the Learning Composite are standard scores (M = 100, SD = 15). CSBS DP scores are standard scores for the composites (M = 10, SD = 3) and Total (M = 100, SD = 15).

p < .001 unless otherwise noted

* p < .01

** p < .05

ns = not significant

and our goal is to improve early identification of these children. Children were classified as *at risk* on the CSBS DP if they performed in the bottom 10th percentile (i.e., a standard score at or below 6 on the composites and 81 on the total).

For the Infant-Toddler Checklist, the criterion for *at risk* was set at performance in the bottom 10th percentile for the Social or Symbolic Composite or Total. Children who were in the bottom 10th percentile on only the Speech Composite were not considered *at risk* because this led to the inclusion of too many late talkers who cleared up; if they also scored low on either the Social or Symbolic Composite, they were more likely to have persisting problems.

For the Caregiver Questionnaire and Behavior Sample, the criterion for *at risk* was set at performance in the bottom 10th percentile for at least one composite and/or the *Total*. The Speech Composite for the Caregiver Questionnaire and Behavior Sample is based on more detailed information than the Infant-Toddler Checklist and was found to provide more precise information about sounds to help predict the late talkers who will have persisting problems.

At follow-up testing, children were classified as having *failed* the Mullen Scales if they performed in the bottom 10th percentile on at least two of the five scales (i.e., Gross Motor, Visual Reception, Fine Motor, Receptive Language, and Expressive Language) or on the Learning Composite *or* in the bottom 2nd percentile on at least one of the five scales.

Agreement between classifications on the CSBS DP and the 2- and 3-year-old follow-up standardized testing are presented in two-way contingency tables in Table 7.24. The following agreement proportions were calculated for each measure to evaluate validity and are reported in Table 7.24:

- *True positives*—the proportion of children identified as at risk (i.e., receiving a positive screen or evaluation result) who failed the follow-up testing; also called sensitivity
- *True negatives*—the proportion of children identified as no risk (i.e., receiving a negative screen or evaluation result) who passed the follow-up testing
- *False positives*—the proportion of children identified as at risk (i.e., receiving a positive screen or evaluation result) who passed the follow-up testing
- *False negatives*—the proportion of children identified as no risk (i.e., receiving a negative screen or evaluation result) who failed the follow-up testing
- *Percent agreement*—the proportion of children correctly identified as either at risk or no risk, based on passing or failing the follow-up testing, respectively
- *Overreferral*—the proportion of children incorrectly identified as at risk out of the total number of children screened or evaluated
- *Underreferral*—the proportion of children incorrectly identified as no risk out of the total number of children screened or evaluated
- *Positive predictive value*—the proportion of children identified as at risk who failed the follow-up testing out of the total number of children identified as at risk.
- *Negative predictive value*—the proportion of children identified as no risk who pass the follow-up testing out of the total number of children identified as no risk.

Table 7.24. Contingency Table for the CSBS DP with the Mullen Scales of Early Learning administered at 2 and 3 years of age

	Infant-Toddler Checklist	Mullen Scales			Caregiver Questionnaire	Mullen Scales			Behavior Sample	Mullen Scales		
		Fail	Pass			Fail	Pass			Fail	Pass	
	Identified at risk	35	26	61	Identified at risk	35	19	54	Identified at risk	32	13	45
	No risk	11	120	131	No risk	5	82	87	No risk	6	90	96
		46	146	192		40	101	141		38	103	141
2-year-old follow-up												
True positives (Sensitivity)	76.1%				87.5%				84.2%			
True negatives (Specificity)	82.2%				81.2%				87.4%			
False positives	17.8%				18.8%				12.6%			
False negatives	23.9%				12.5%				15.8%			
Percent agreement	80.7%				83.0%				86.5%			
Overreferral	13.5%				13.5%				9.2%			
Underreferral	5.7%				3.6%				4.3%			
Positive predictive value	57.4%				64.8%				71.1%			
Negative predictive value	91.6%				94.3%				93.8%			
	Infant-Toddler Checklist				**Caregiver Questionnaire**				**Behavior Sample**			
		Fail	Pass			Fail	Pass			Fail	Pass	
	Identified at risk	16	20	36	Identified at risk	14	10	24	Identified at risk	16	11	27
	No risk	3	53	56	No risk	4	63	67	No risk	3	60	63
		19	73	92		18	73	91		19	71	90
3-year-old follow-up												
True positives (Sensitivity)	84.2%				77.8%				84.2%			
True negatives (Specificity)	72.6%				86.3%				84.5%			
False positives	27.4%				13.7%				15.5%			
False negatives	15.8%				22.2%				15.8%			
Percent agreement	75.0%				84.6%				84.4%			
Overreferral	21.7%				11.0%				12.2%			
Underreferral	3.3%				4.4%				3.3%			
Positive predictive value	44.4%				58.3%				59.3%			
Negative predictive value	94.6%				94.0%				95.2%			

These results provide good evidence for the predictive validity of all three components of the CSBS DP. Agreement proportions for the Infant-Toddler Checklist indicate good validity for a brief screening measure. Agreement proportions for the Caregiver Questionnaire and Behavior Sample are fairly comparable, and both are better than the Infant-Toddler Checklist, which is to be expected given the brevity of the Infant-Toddler Checklist. These findings support the use of the Caregiver Questionnaire and the Behavior Sample as a second-level evaluation following the Infant-Toddler Checklist. All three components show fairly similar agreement proportions from the 2- to the 3-year-old follow-up testing. These agreement proportions are based on criterion testing that ranges from 4–11 months later at the 2-year-old follow-up testing and 18–22 months later at the 3-year-old follow-up testing. This is particularly noteworthy because the agreement proportions are comparable or better in comparison with what other instruments have documented for concurrent validity (i.e., based on comparison with other measures gathered at the same time) with infants and toddlers.

In conclusion, these validation studies demonstrate that the CSBS DP is effective at measuring early prelinguistic communication skills and predicting a child's relative performance on measures 1–2 years later. These findings strongly support the predictive validity of the CSBS DP Infant-Toddler Checklist, CSBS DP Caregiver Questionnaire, and CSBS DP Behavior Sample and the use of a collection of prelinguistic measures, rather than the use of words alone, to improve the accuracy of early identification of very young children. However, it is important to be aware of the inaccuracy of all three components. That is, on the parent report measures, a small proportion of parents overestimate or underestimate their children's abilities. On the face-to-face evaluation, a small proportion of children perform below their potential or the measure does not detect a small proportion of children who will have later learning problems. It is for this reason that we designed the CSBS DP to utilize multiple sources of information and that we strongly recommend using a combination of parent report and face-to-face evaluation procedures with very young children.

8 INTERPRETING RESULTS

This chapter describes how to interpret the results for each of the three components of the CSBS DP: the Infant-Toddler Checklist, the Caregiver Questionnaire, and the Behavior Sample. The first part of the chapter describes general issues for interpreting all three components of the CSBS DP. The next part addresses screening decisions based on the Infant-Toddler Checklist and provides guidelines for writing an Infant-Toddler Checklist: Screening Report. The last part of the chapter addresses evaluation decisions based on the Caregiver Questionnaire and Behavior Sample and provides guidelines for clinical report writing.

GENERAL ISSUES FOR INTERPRETING THE CSBS DP

The reliability and validity findings reported in Chapter 7 support the use of the CSBS DP as a screening and evaluation tool with children 6–24 months of age. The CSBS DP maximizes the role of the family in evaluation by using cost-efficient parent report tools. In addition, parents are present and participate in the face-to-face evaluation, which reflects family-centered practices as mandated for infants and toddlers by the Individuals with Disabilities Education Act (IDEA) Amendments of 1997 (PL 105-17).

Another advantage of the CSBS DP is that standard scores and percentiles are available for all three measures, whereas most screening tools report only pass/fail cutoff scores. Normative scores allow service providers to decide the cutoff based on state eligibility requirements and to monitor more carefully children who fall between the 10th and 25th percentiles. Eligibility criteria for early intervention services through Part C of the IDEA Amendments of 1997 (PL 105-17) vary from state to state, ranging from 1 to 2 standard deviations (SDs) below the mean; however, to improve early identification of children with developmental disabilities, eligibility criteria that will catch a sensible proportion of children must be used. Because 10%– 15% of school-age children have disabilities, we recommend a cutoff of at least 1.25 SD below the mean, which corresponds with the bottom 10th percentile. This will allow earlier identification of the majority of children who will require special education at school age. Setting the cutoff at 2 SDs below the mean, which corresponds with the bottom 2nd percentile, will continue to miss most of the children who will require special education when they get to school age.

The accuracy and effectiveness of parent report compared with face-to-face evaluation are difficult to determine with very young children. There are advantages and limitations of both evaluation methods. Parent report can be inaccurate if parents over- or underestimate their children's abilities. The strength of the relationship between the CSBS DP's parent report tools and the face-to-face evaluation (as reported in Chapter 7) suggests a moderate to high degree of accuracy, similar to the research findings with other parent report tools (Fenson et al., 1993; Rescorla & Alley, 2001;

Squires, Potter, & Bricker, 1999); however, there is still a degree of inaccuracy with parent report. Therefore, it is important to use a parent report tool with caution and sound clinical judgment so that parents are not needlessly concerned. The three measures of the CSBS DP can be used in combination so that a clinical decision is based on both parent report and face-to-face evaluation.

One possible way to increase the accuracy of parent report is to use more than one parent report tool. The *Ages & Stages Questionnaires: A Parent Completed, Child-Monitoring System* (2nd ed., ASQ, Squires et al., 1999) is a widely used child-monitoring system, which, like the CSBS DP Infant-Toddler Checklist, uses parent report as a method to screen young children. The ASQ has 19 questionnaires from 4 months to 60 months, linked to specific ages (e.g., 12-month questionnaire). Each questionnaire includes six questions in five domains and has pass/fail cutoff points. We recommend using the ASQ along with the CSBS DP Infant-Toddler Checklist or as a follow-up with the CSBS DP Caregiver Questionnaire because the questionnaires provide complementary information.

Parent report is ineffective if parents do not complete and return the evaluation tool. Research on parent report tools reveals that a large percentage of parents do not return questionnaires received in the mail. Sixty-four percent of families do not return forms when they are not contacted ahead of time (Fenson et al., 1993), and twenty-five percent to forty percent of families do not return forms even if they are contacted ahead of time and agree to return the questionnaires (Fenson et al., 1993; Rescorla & Alley, 2001; Wetherby, Allen, Cleary, Kublin, & Goldstein, 2001). Therefore, when using parent report for screening and evaluation, it is important to plan follow-up methods if questionnaires are mailed to families. We find the Infant-Toddler Checklist to be most effective if completed by families on site when distributed at a health care or child care facility, rather than taken home and returned in the mail.

Although parents may over- or underestimate their child's abilities with parent report tools, it is challenging to secure accurate measures of abilities in very young children based on face-to-face evaluations. Many factors may influence children's performance, including attention, interest, fatigue, comfort level, and experience being in unfamiliar settings. The naturalistic sampling procedures of the CSBS DP Behavior Sample were designed to put the child and parent at ease and encourage communication. Having the parent present and asking the parent to participate during the Behavior Sample should increase the likelihood of gathering a representative sample and provide a context to build consensus with the parent about the child's strengths and weaknesses.

A face-to-face evaluation may be limited in effectiveness because families may not agree to participate in an evaluation or may not show up for a scheduled evaluation. We recommend using a combination of parent report and face-to-face evaluation to offer families both methods. For families who choose to participate in both, this provides the opportunity to look for a convergence of findings from multiple sources of information, and if the findings are discrepant, to explore reasons why they are so.

Socioeconomic Class

A limitation of the normative sample for the CSBS DP is the under-representation of families of lower socioeconomic status (SES). Families of minority ethnicities were more likely to complete the Infant-Toddler Checklist than to complete either the Caregiver Questionnaire or the Behavior Sample, but only a small proportion of families of lower SES participated in the normative sample. The age and education level of the families participating in the normative sample are very similar to normative samples with other standardized evaluation tools for young children (e.g., Fenson et al., 1993; Mullen, 1995).

Extreme caution is needed in using the CSBS DP and other screening and evaluation tools with families of lower SES if they are not well represented in the normative sample. In studies of social class with the MacArthur Communication Development Inventory (CDI; Fenson et al., 1993), there were significant differences in word comprehension on the Words and Gestures section and in vocabulary production on the Words and Sentences section for children 20 months of age and younger. With the CDI, parents of lower SES tended to check more items on the inventories than parents of higher SES. These findings suggest that parents with less education may overestimate their children's language abilities and that parents with more education may underestimate their children's language abilities. When administering the CSBS DP parent report tools with a parent who has less than a high school education, a service provider should go over the information in a face-to-face meeting with the parent to ensure that the parent understands the questions. It is important to consider ways to offer developmental screening and evaluation so that a greater number of families from diverse cultures and SES levels will participate.

Ceiling and Floor Effects

As commonly found with standardized tools, there are ceiling and floor effects with the components of the CSBS DP. It is important for evaluators to be aware of these and to use this information in interpreting results. A ceiling effect is when a large proportion of children in a normative age group is achieving the maximum possible score. A floor effect is when a large proportion of children in a normative age group is achieving the minimum possible score. A ceiling or floor effect is evident to a small extent for the total and composite scores and to a greater extent for some of the cluster scores. The norms tables for each component reveal where ceiling and floor effects exist.

A ceiling effect is evident if the highest possible raw score spans across several standard scores (and corresponding percentiles) for a particular age. In creating the norms tables, if a raw score fell across several different standard scores, we assigned the raw score to the highest one. Thus, the cells in the norms tables are blank if there were repeated raw scores. Refer to the norms tables for the Infant-Toddler Checklist in Appendix A. For example, a 24-month-old child who earned a raw score of 26 on the Social Composite of the Infant-Toddler Checklist has a standard score ranging from 13 to 17 and a percentile rank ranging from 84 to 99. This child would be assigned a standard score of 17 and a percentile rank of 99 because it is the highest score and a conservative estimate of this child's relative standing in the group, but that child could be functioning as low as the 84th percentile.

Continue to refer to the norms table for the Infant-Toddler Checklist in Appendix A to identify ceiling effects. For the Social Composite of the CSBS DP

Infant-Toddler Checklist, there is a very slight ceiling effect beginning at 12 months of age, which becomes more prominent at 21 months. What this means is that the Infant-Toddler Checklist does not differentiate between children who perform between the 84th and 99th percentiles at 24 months. For the Speech and Symbolic Composites and the Total there is also a very slight ceiling effect beginning at about 14 months of age, which becomes more prominent at 21 months. The largest ceiling effect found on the Infant-Toddler Checklist is on the Speech and Symbolic Composites at 22–24 months of age. The highest possible score of 14 on the Speech Composite and 17 on the Symbolic Composite corresponds with a standard score ranging from 12 to 17 and percentile ranging from 75 to 99.

Similar patterns in ceiling effects are also evident on the norms tables for the Caregiver Questionnaire and the Behavior Sample and are more pronounced for some of the cluster scores than for the composite scores or total score. Refer to the norms tables for the Caregiver Questionnaire. The largest ceiling effect found on the Caregiver Questionnaire is on the Gestures Cluster at 19–24 months. The highest possible score of 12 corresponds with a standard score ranging from 10 to 17 and percentile ranging from 50 to 99. This means that by 19 months of age one could expect about half of the children to get all 12 points on the Gestures Cluster.

Refer to the norms tables for the Behavior Sample in Appendix A. It is interesting to note that there is not a ceiling effect on the Gestures Cluster of the Behavior Sample. The largest ceiling effect found on the Behavior Sample is on the Understanding Cluster at 21–24 months of age. The highest possible score of 24 corresponds with a standard score ranging from 11 to 17 and percentile ranging from 63 to 99. There is also a large ceiling effect for the Understanding Cluster of the Caregiver Questionnaire.

For clinical use of the CSBS DP, a ceiling effect is not problematic because the tool is intended to precisely identify children who fall at the bottom end of the normative tables. In fact, it can offer more confidence in expectations that children should be able to perform the skills that are being measured. When a large ceiling effect exists, caution should be taken in interpreting a child's score as above average versus average. Other tools that are more precise measures of language at the older age range should be used in combination with the CSBS DP. A ceiling effect may be problematic for research studies using correlational analyses because there will be a restricted range where there is a ceiling effect; however, the extent of the ceiling effect was not problematic for the studies that we have conducted and reported in this manual. Using the composites instead of the clusters will reduce the extent of the ceiling effect.

A floor effect is evident if the lowest possible score spans across several standard scores (and corresponding percentiles) for a particular age. As noted previously, in creating the norms tables, if a raw score fell across several different standard scores, we assigned the raw score to the highest one, which may overestimate an individual child's relative performance. Floor effects are not evident on the CSBS DP Infant-Toddler Checklist norms but are evident on both the Caregiver Questionnaire and Behavior Sample. Refer to the norms tables for the Caregiver Questionnaire and Behavior Sample in Appendix A to identify floor effects.

The largest floor effect found on both the Caregiver Questionnaire and the Behavior Sample is on the Words Cluster at the youngest age ranges because most children do not use words until at least 12 months of age, and some children still do not use words until at least 18 months of age. The largest floor effect found on the Caregiver Questionnaire is on the Words Cluster at 6–7 months. A score of 0 corresponds with a standard score ranging from 3 to 14 and a percentile ranging from 1 to 91. This means that at 6 months of age, one would expect about 91% of children to use no words and get a 0 on the Words Cluster. Assigning a child to the 91st percentile means that this child's performance is anywhere between the 1st and 91st percentiles. In other words, this cluster does not differentiate among children between the 1st to the 91st percentiles at 6–7 months of age.

Similarly, the largest floor effect found on the Behavior Sample is on the Words Cluster at 12–14 months of age. A score of 0 corresponds with a standard score ranging from 3 to 10 and a percentile ranging from the 1st to the 50th. In other words, about half of 12- to 14-month-olds use no words during the sample; therefore, this response would be considered average. A small number of these children will likely end up in the bottom 10th percentile on the Words Cluster when they are older, but it cannot be determined which children will from their performance on this cluster at this age.

For clinical use of the CSBS DP, a floor effect can be problematic. The standard scores and percentiles from the norms tables may indicate that a child is functioning in the average or above average range when the child is in the concern range. If a floor effect is present, this means that the particular score is not precise at that age range. This fact needs to be considered in the interpretation and reporting of the results. Therefore, users need to understand the floor effects and be extremely careful in interpreting standard scores and percentiles when there is a floor effect. Children need to be followed past the age range of the floor effect to get more precise measures of these skills. A floor effect may be problematic for research studies using correlational analyses, similar to ceiling effects, because there will be a restricted range where there is a floor effect; however, the extent of the floor effect was not problematic for the studies that we have conducted and reported in this manual.

Because of the potential problems associated with floor effects, we recommend that only the Composite and Total Scores for the Caregiver Questionnaire and Behavior Sample be reported to families. The only floor effects are on the Speech Composite for both the Caregiver Questionnaire and the Behavior Sample for the youngest age groups. At these earlier ages, the Social and Symbolic Composites are more precise measures. The cluster scores can be used to better understand children's weaknesses, but caution should be used in interpreting strengths if there are floor effects.

Children Older than 24 Months of Age

The norms for the CSBS DP only go through 24 months of age. The components of the CSBS DP can be used with children older than 24 months of age as long as they are functioning below a 24-month age level. A child older than 24 months of age can be compared with the oldest age group for each of the components (i.e., 24 months for the Infant-Toddler Checklist, 23–24 months for the Caregiver Questionnaire, and 21–24 months for the Behavior Sample); however, the evaluator needs to be very careful in interpreting and reporting standard scores and percentiles. If any of the child's scores fall above the concern range (i.e., above the 10th percentile), the evaluator cannot be confident that the child is performing as expected for his or her age because the CSBS DP does not interpret whether children older than 24 months would score even higher on these measures. In other words, the standard scores and percentiles may be overestimating the child's true performance because they are comparing that child with a younger normative group.

For example, if an evaluator uses the Infant-Toddler Checklist with a 26-month-old child and the child scores in the 16th percentile or higher on all composites, the evaluator should *not* send a report indicating that the child is performing as expected for his or her age. Rather, he or she needs to inform the parents that the child is too old to use the norms for this tool. If the same child scores at the 9th percentile, it would be appropriate to refer the child for an evaluation; however, it is important to only report that the child is performing in the bottom 10th percentile and not to report the specific percentile because that child may actually be performing lower than the 9th percentile when compared with children of the same age. Keep in mind that if the child is performing in the bottom 10th percentile, we recommend that evaluators do not report the specific percentile to parents, even for children younger than 24 months (see sample reports in next section).

Similarly, for the Caregiver Questionnaire and Behavior Sample, if any of the child's scores fall above the concern range (i.e., above the 10th percentile), the evaluator cannot be confident that the child is performing as expected for his or her age, particularly if the child is performing at the 16th or even 25th percentile. If any of the child's scores fall below the concern range (i.e., in the bottom 10th percentile), this would indicate that the child is performing below age expectations; however, it is better to report that the child is performing in the bottom 10th percentile, rather than reporting specific standard scores and percentiles because the standard scores and percentiles based on 24-month-olds may be overestimating the performance of an older child.

SCREENING DECISIONS BASED ON THE INFANT-TODDLER CHECKLIST

The Infant-Toddler Checklist is a first step in routine developmental screening for children 6–24 months of age to decide if a developmental evaluation is needed. The scoring decisions for the Infant-Toddler Checklist are provided in Chapter 3. A service provider may use the Infant-Toddler Checklist without using the other components of the CSBS DP. If a child is referred for a developmental evaluation using more traditional evaluation tools that measure receptive and expressive language, as a follow-up to the Checklist, it is possible that there will not be agreement because the Checklist is measuring different skills. Because the CSBS DP measures social and symbolic aspects of communication and language development, it may identify children as at risk who may perform better on more traditional tests that only measure vocabulary or structural aspects of language. This phenomenon can be confusing to families, so it is important that users of the Infant-Toddler Checklist understand the domains that it measures.

The Infant-Toddler Checklist should be used to monitor development about every 3 months between 6 and 24 months. Because it is based on parent report, it is possible for the caregiver to overestimate or underestimate the child's abilities. Therefore, this tool should be used along with a brief observation of the child by a health care or child care service provider. The Infant-Toddler Checklist should only be used to decide that further information or a developmental evaluation is needed. Caution should be taken not to alarm parents. We find that many parents already have concerns about their child, especially as their child is approaching about 18 months of age and is behind in language development. As noted previously, the early intervention literature emphasizes the notion of multiple risk factors; therefore, a child's scores on the Infant-Toddler Checklist need to be considered in relation to other known biological or environmental risk factors. Clinical judgment should be used in making decisions about the need for further evaluation with the standard scores as guidelines. Remember that the Infant-Toddler Checklist is not meant for a developmental or diagnostic evaluation and should not be used to determine if a child has a developmental delay or to make a differential diagnosis.

Guidelines for Reporting the Infant-Toddler Checklist Results

We have developed two report formats for the CSBS DP Infant-Toddler Checklist, which should be sent out within 1 week of receiving the Checklist. One is the Infant-Toddler Checklist: Screening Report, which includes the child's raw scores, standard scores, and percentiles ranks and is placed in the child's health record. The other is a letter to parents that summarizes the recommendation based on the Infant-Toddler Checklist results. The letter to parents does not include scores but briefly explains what the Checklist measures, whether a developmental evaluation is recommended, and if so, why this evaluation is important.

We have developed three different versions of the letter to parents based on the recommendation made. The first letter is for children who perform in the no concern range on all three composites and indicates that the child is currently communicating as expected for his or her age and that the child should be monitored with another Checklist in 3 months (see Figure 8.1). The second letter is for children who perform in the concern range on the Speech Composite only for the first time and recommends that the child should be monitored with another Checklist in 3 months (see Figure 8.2). The third letter is for children who perform in the concern range on the Social and/or Symbolic Composite and recommends referring the child for a developmental evaluation (see Figure 8.3).

Examples of the letter to parents and Infant-Toddler Checklist: Screening Report for a sample child, Casey, are included in Figures 8.4 and 8.5. The information reported by Casey's mother on the Infant-Toddler Checklist indicates that he is in the concern range on the Speech and Symbolic Composites; therefore, a developmental evaluation is recommended. The wording of these reports should be used as a model for reporting information from the Infant-Toddler Checklist. These reports can be generated and printed with the **CSBS DP Infant-Toddler Checklist and Easy-Score** CD-Rom and User's Guide.

EVALUATION DECISIONS BASED ON THE CAREGIVER QUESTIONNAIRE AND BEHAVIOR SAMPLE

The second step in the CSBS DP two-step process is evaluating with the Caregiver Questionnaire and Behavior Sample. Scoring decisions for the CSBS DP Caregiver

Re: CSBS DP™ **Infant-Toddler Checklist**

Child's name: ______________________

Date of birth: ______________________

Date Checklist completed: ______________

Chronological age (in months): __________

Referral recommended: No

Dear (parent's name):

Thank you for taking the time to complete the *Infant-Toddler Checklist*. The Checklist was used to screen your child's ability to communicate using eye gaze, gestures, sounds, or words and to play with toys.

Based on the information you provided on the Checklist, your child is currently communicating as expected for his or her age. Because new skills are emerging each month, it is important to monitor (child's name)'s development, and we would like you to complete the Checklist again in about 3 months.

We will contact you at the appropriate time to provide you with a Checklist. If you have any questions or concerns about your child's development, please feel free to call us.

We look forward to assisting you.

Sincerely,

(Examiner's name)

Figure 8.1. Letter to parents with referral not recommended.

Re: CSBS DP Infant-Toddler Checklist

Child's name: ______________________

Date of birth: ______________________

Date Checklist completed: ______________

Chronological age (in months): __________

Referral recommended: Not Yet

Dear (parent's name):

Thank you for taking the time to complete the *Infant-Toddler Checklist*. The Checklist was used to screen your child's ability to communicate using eye gaze, gestures, sounds, or words and to play with toys.

Based on the information you provided on the Checklist, we are recommending that your child's development be monitored so we can see how (child's name)'s skills are emerging. We would like you to complete the Checklist again in about 3 months.

We will contact you at the appropriate time to provide you with a Checklist. If you have any questions or concerns about your child's development, please feel free to call us.

We look forward to assisting you.

Sincerely,

(Examiner's name)

Figure 8.2. Letter to parents with referral not yet recommended.

Re: CSBS DP™ **Infant-Toddler Checklist**

Child's name: ______________________

Date of birth: ______________________

Date Checklist completed: ____________

Chronological age (in months): ________

Referral recommended: Yes

Dear (parent's name):

Thank you for taking the time to complete the *Infant-Toddler Checklist*. The Checklist was used to screen (child's name)'s ability to communicate using eye gaze, gestures, sounds, or words and to play with toys.

Based on the information you provided on the Checklist, we are recommending that (child's name) be referred for a developmental evaluation. Please call our office so we can help make these arrangements.

The Checklist does not conclusively determine if your child has a problem in development, but indicates whether further evaluation or follow-up is needed. A more thorough developmental evaluation can determine if (child's name) has a communication delay. If needed, we will provide information for planning the next steps to support you and your child. Children who have early communication delays may have difficulties in other areas of development. It is important to catch communication problems in young children as early as possible, as early intervention services may remediate or lessen the impact of communication problems and help you support your child's development.

We look forward to assisting you.

Sincerely,

(Examiner's name)

Figure 8.3. Letter to parents with referral recommended.

Re: CSBS DP Infant-Toddler Checklist

Child's name: Casey Smith

Date of birth: May 17, 2000

Date Checklist completed: January 25, 2002

Chronological age (in months): 20 months

Referral recommended: Yes

Dear Ms. Smith:

Thank you for taking the time to complete the *Infant-Toddler Checklist*. The Checklist was used to screen Casey's ability to communicate using eye gaze, gestures, sounds, or words and to play with toys.

Based on the information you provided on the Checklist, we are recommending that Casey be referred for a developmental evaluation. Please call our office so we can help make these arrangements.

The Checklist does not conclusively determine if your child has a problem in development but indicates whether further evaluation or follow-up is needed. A more thorough developmental evaluation can determine if Casey has a communication delay. If needed, we will provide information for planning the next steps to support you and your child. Children who have early communication delays may have difficulties in other areas of development. It is important to catch communication problems in young children as early as possible, as early intervention services may remediate or lessen the impact of communication problems and help you support your child's development.

We look forward to assisting you.

Sincerely,

Jane Miller, M.S., CCC-SLP

Figure 8.4. Letter to parents for Casey.

CSBS DP Infant-Toddler Checklist: Screening Report

Child's name: Casey

Date filled out: 1/25/02

Date of birth: 5/17/00

Chronological age[1]***:*** 20

[1] If child is 4 or more weeks premature, use corrected age. Calculate chronological age by subtracting Date of birth from Date the Checklist was filled out.

Checklist Results

Predictor	Raw Score		Standard Score[a,b]	Percentile Rank[b]	Concern[c]
Emotion and Eye Gaze	8				
Communication	6				
Gestures	8				
SOCIAL COMPOSITE		22	9	37	
Sounds	5				
Words	0				
SPEECH COMPOSITE		5	4	2	Yes
Understanding	4				
Object Use	7				
SYMBOLIC COMPOSITE		11	6	9	Yes
TOTAL		38	81	10	Yes

[a] The standard scores are based on a mean of 10 and SD of 3 for the Composite Scores and a mean of 100 and SD of 15 for the Total Score. (Refer to the *CSBS DP Manual, First Normed Edition*, for standard scores and tables of norms.)

[b] Criterion levels for concern are set at more than 1.25 SD below the mean as follows: Standard Scores at or below 6 for the Composite Scores and 81 for the Total Score; Percentiles at or below 10. (Refer to the *CSBS DP Manual, First Normed Edition,* for standard scores, percentiles, and tables of norms.)

[c] After filling in Standard Score and Percentile Rank, if below criterion level, write *Yes* in the Concern box. If at or above criterion level, leave blank. A child should be referred for an evaluation if the Social Composite, Symbolic Composite, *or* the Total Score is below criterion level. A child should be monitored carefully if the Speech Composite is below criterion level; administer a Checklist again in 3 months, and if the child's scores remain below criterion level, refer for a developmental evaluation.

Recommendation

Based on the information provided on the Infant-Toddler Checklist and the results shown above, the following recommendation is made at this time (check one):

- ☐ This child currently communicates as expected for his or her age. Because new skills are emerging each month, it is important to monitor this child's development by asking the child's caregiver to complete the Checklist again in 3 months.
- ☐ This child should be carefully monitored. Re-administer the Checklist in 3 months to determine if a developmental evaluation will become advisable.
- ☒ This child should be referred for a developmental evaluation.

Figure 8.5. Infant-Toddler Checklist: Screening Report for Casey.

Questionnaire are presented in Chapter 4. Scoring decisions for the CSBS DP Behavior Sample are presented in Chapter 5. The Caregiver Questionnaire is based on parent report, and, as with the Checklist, it is possible for the caregiver to overestimate or underestimate the child's abilities. The Behavior Sample is based on a face-to-face evaluation, and it is possible to underestimate the child's abilities because the child may be apprehensive, anxious, shy, uninterested, or uncooperative. The Behavior Sample: Caregiver Perception Rating Form completed by the parent after the Behavior Sample can help determine whether the child behaved typically during the Behavior Sample. We recommend that these two components be used together. If a consistent pattern of concerns is documented on the Caregiver Questionnaire and Behavior Sample, the child should be referred for a diagnostic evaluation and/or for further assessment to plan support or intervention services. If there is a discrepancy between the pattern of scores on the Caregiver Questionnaire and the Behavior Sample, reasons for this discrepancy should be considered (i.e., Is the parent over- or underestimating the child's performance or is the child performing below potential on the Behavior Sample?). While these components can be used independently, we recommend using them together to increase the accuracy of the evaluation information and to build consensus with the family.

The Caregiver Questionnaire and the Behavior Sample should only be used to decide whether a child has developmental delays. They are not meant for a diagnostic evaluation and should not be used as the only source of information for a differential diagnosis. Caution should be taken not to alarm parents. As noted previously, many parents already have concerns about their child. Clinical judgment should be used in making decisions about the need for further evaluation with the cutoffs provided in Chapters 4 and 5 as guidelines.

Some children perform poorly on the CSBS DP but perform well on other standardized tests. This may reflect inaccuracies in measurement but also may reflect differences in what the tests are measuring. The CSBS DP measures social and communication skills that are not measured on most standardized tests. Children who have social-communicative problems, such as children with autism spectrum disorders, would be expected to have scores in the concern range on the Social Composite and possibly the Symbolic Composite. Children with social-communicative problems who are higher functioning and are beginning to use words may score within normal limits on standardized tests of receptive and expressive language at a young age. A child should not automatically be suspected of having autism spectrum disorder if his or her scores on the Social Composite indicate cause for concern. Children with other developmental delays may also score low on the Social Composite; however, if a child does score low on the Social Composite, the clinician should consider whether the child shows any characteristics of an autism spectrum disorder and refer the child for a diagnostic evaluation.

In addition, some children perform well on the CSBS DP but perform poorly on other standardized tests. Again, this may reflect inaccuracies in measurement but also may reflect differences in what the tests are measuring. Because the CSBS DP measures social and communication skills, children who have mild speech-language delays may not score in the concern range (i.e., bottom 10th percentile), even on the Speech Composite. Because of the floor effect, a child cannot score in the concern range on the Speech Composite until at least 15 months of age. Research on prelinguistic predictors reviewed in Chapter 2 suggests that children who will have persisting language delays will be low on skills measured in the Social and Symbolic Composites at young ages.

Children in the 21- to 24-month age range who have only a few words may score in the bottom 16th percentile and not the bottom 10th percentile on the Speech Composite for the Caregiver Questionnaire and Behavior Sample. The reason for this is that at least 15% of 24-month-old children are late talkers. Two parent report tools that are widely used and provide more detailed information about vocabulary production in 2-year-olds are the MacArthur CDI/Words and Sentences (Fenson et al., 1993) and the Language Development Survey (LDS; Rescorla and Alley, 2001). Any child who performs in the bottom 16th percentile on the Speech Composite on either the Caregiver Questionnaire or the Behavior Sample should be given the CDI or the LDS as a follow-up. The CDI/Words and Sentences is normed from 16 to 30 months of age. The LDS is briefer, and norms are available at 24 months of age. Further speech and language testing may also be recommended based on clinical judgment.

Feedback After the Behavior Sample

When a parent brings a child in for a face-to-face evaluation, the clinician should give the parent feedback about how the child performed during the Behavior Sample. Because the Behavior Sample may be scored later from a videotape, the clinician may need to provide this feedback before actually scoring the sample. Following are guidelines for providing feedback on the CSBS DP Behavior Sample. Make sure to review the CSBS DP Infant-Toddler Checklist and CSBS DP Caregiver Questionnaire before meeting the family so that you can refer to the information that the parent already provided when you talk with him or her during the Behavior Sample and feedback session. It can be helpful to have the child's file with the parent report tools in it to glance at during the feedback.

The feedback should consist of a brief review of how the child did in each of the seven cluster areas. Table 8.1 provides developmental guidelines that may be helpful during the feedback. This table is based on raw scores and includes average and expected raw scores for each of the 20 items measured during the Behavior Sample for each of the four age groups. The average is based on what 50% of the children in the normative sample did (i.e., the 50th percentile), and the expected is based on what 80% of the children did (i.e., the 20th percentile).

As the clinician becomes more familiar with the sampling and scoring procedures, he or she can keep track of what the child did during the Behavior Sample and whether the child is in the average range or at least is above the expected range. The clinician can use the average range to let parents know what is typical behavior at their child's age and what skills to expect their child to develop in the next few months. If the child does not display the number of skills that is expected, then the clinician can alert the parent of these concern areas. It is important to be aware that these raw scores reflect what children in the normative sample did during the Behavior Sample and that parents may report higher numbers on the Caregiver Questionnaire. In addition, children may use higher rates of behaviors in familiar settings. For example, at least 50% of the children age 21–24 months in the CSBS DP normative sample used 11 different words during the Behavior Sample. Because the

Table 8.1. CSBS DP Behavior Sample milestones

	12–14 months		15–17 months		18–20 months		21–24 months		Total score
	Average 50%	Expected 80%	Average 50%	Expected 80%	Average 50%	Expected 80%	Average 50%	Expected 80%	
Emotion and Eye Gaze									
1. Gaze shifts	6	5	6	5	6	5	6	5	6
2. Shared positive affect	4	2	4	2	4	2	4	2	6
3. Gaze/point following	2	0	2	1	2	1	2	2	2
Communication									
4. Rate of communication	18	15	18	15	18	16	18	17	18
5. Behavior regulation	6	5	6	5	6	5	6	5	6
6. Social interaction	1	0	1	0	2	0	3	1	6
7. Joint attention	4	1	4	2	5	3	5	3	6
Gestures									
8. Inventory of conventional gestures	5	3	5	3	5	4	6	4	8
9. Distal gestures	4	2	4	2	5	3	5	3	6
Sounds									
10. Syllables with consonants	4	1	4	2	6	4	6	4	6
11. Inventory of consonants	3	1	4	2	5	3	6	3	10
Words									
12. Words	0	0	2	0	4	1	6	3	6
13. Inventory of words	0	0	2	0	5	1	11	3	16
14. Word combinations	0	0	0	0	0	0	1	0	6
15. Inventory of word combinations	0	0	0	0	0	0	2	0	8
Understanding									
16. Language comprehension	1	0	3	1	5	2	7	4	8
Object Use									
17. Inventory of action schemes	5	3	6	4	7	5	7	6	12
18. Action schemes to other	1	0	2	1	3	2	3	2	6
19. Action schemes in sequence	0	0	1	0	2	1	2	1	6
20. Stacks tower of blocks	2	1	3	2	4	2	5	4	5

CSBS DP Behavior Sample is only a brief sample of the child's behavior, these results do not mean that an average child at this age only has 11 words in his or her vocabulary. In fact, the parents of the children in the normative sample reported that their children used a larger number of words at home.

CASEY: 21 MONTHS

Following is an example of information that the clinician provided for Casey's mother based on his Behavior Sample:

"The areas I was looking for during this evaluation are the same as those you reported on when you completed the longer questionnaire last month. The first area I looked at is Casey's ability to use eye gaze to communicate with you and smile to share pleasure. This is one of the fundamental parts of communication because a child has to learn to look at the person he is communicating with. It is also important that he looks at your eyes and looks back and forth between toys and your eyes to share his observations with you. You reported that Casey often looks at you when playing with toys at home, and I noticed that he did this frequently during this evaluation. It was also nice the way he smiled at you when the two of you were playing with the dog toy.

Next, I looked at how Casey communicates. At Casey's age, I would expect that he would be able to communicate for three basic reasons or purposes. First, children communicate to ask for help. I noticed this when Casey gave you the jar of bubbles to get you to blow them. Second, children communicate to get your attention. We often see this when children play Peekaboo, tug on you to get you to look, and wave hello and bye-bye. I saw Casey wave bye-bye to the toys when I removed them and then look over at you. Third, children communicate to get you to look at things that they have or to share what they are focused on. Casey did this several times today, including showing you the dog toy. It's great that Casey was able to communicate for all three reasons during the sample.

Next, I looked at how Casey uses gestures to communicate. Children usually communicate first with gestures and then add sounds to gestures, which helps them begin to use words. Casey used a nice variety of gestures today; he gave you the wind-up toy, waved bye-bye, showed the dog toy, and shook his head "no." I didn't see him point today; is that something you have seen him do?

Next, I looked at how Casey uses sounds. At Casey's age, children usually use about six different consonants including early sounds such as /m/, /b/, /d/, and /g/. I noticed that Casey used the /b/ sound today, and you're reporting that he's using the /b/, /d/, and /g/ sounds at home. Are there any new sounds he's trying? Does he use these sounds often? Is he usually quiet or does he make sounds often?

I also looked at whether Casey uses words. At Casey's age, children usually use about 10 different words during the sample. I didn't hear him use any words today, and you reported that he is not yet using words at home. Are there any new words he is trying?

Next, I looked at his understanding of words. A child usually understands some words before saying words. Casey did a nice job identifying body parts and familiar people today. Do you notice that he seems to follow simple directions at home? Casey didn't give me the objects when I named them, but that sometimes happens with very young children. Does he do this at home?

The last thing I looked at was play. I looked at Casey's play because the way he plays can tell me about his language development. Typically, when children begin to use objects functionally, they begin to use their first words. Then, they learn to play with toys toward someone else like a baby doll or stuffed animal as they begin to develop a little bit larger vocabulary. Then, as they begin to combine play actions, for example stirring with the spoon and feeding Big Bird, they typically begin to imitate or use two-word phrases. Casey used a few actions with the toys, but less than most children his age. He also did not seem very interested in these toys, so that may be why he did not show much play. He did stack five blocks, which is good for his age.

Based on what you reported and what I saw here today, it seems that Casey is communicating a little below what I would expect for a child his age. He is still very young, so I am encouraged that he will make good progress in the next few months. Since you expressed concern about Casey's delay in language development, you may be interested in beginning language intervention. We also offer toddler playgroups. They are designed to give you the opportunity to learn how to encourage communication development; you can ask questions, and you will have time to focus on how to play with Casey."

SAMANTHA: 13 MONTHS

Following is an example of information that the clinician provided for Samantha. It illustrates feedback provided for a mother of a younger child based on the Behavior Sample.

"The areas I was looking for during this evaluation are the same as those you reported on when you completed the longer questionnaire last month. The first area I looked at was Samantha's ability to use eye gaze to communicate with you and to smile at you to share pleasure. This is one of the fundamental parts of communication because a child has to learn to look at the person she is communicating with. It is also important that she looks at your eyes and looks back and forth between toys and your eyes to share her observations with you. You reported that Samantha sometimes looks at you when playing with toys at home, and I noticed that she did this a few times during this evaluation. It was also nice the way she smiled and squealed when she saw the bubbles, but I didn't see her look at you to see if you were sharing the fun with her. Does she do that at home?

Next, I looked at how Samantha communicates. At Samantha's age, I would expect that she would be able to communicate for three basic reasons or purposes. First, children communicate to ask for help. I noticed this when Samantha gave you the jar of bubbles to get you to blow them. Second, children communicate to get your attention. We often see this when children play Peekaboo, tug on you to get you to look, and wave hello and bye-bye. I didn't see Samantha trying to get your attention during the sample. Third, children communicate to get you to look at things that they have or to share what they are focused on. One time Samantha held the wind-up toy out toward you and then pulled it back, maybe to get you to look at it. I didn't see her show you objects any other times. Samantha should be communicating frequently for all three reasons in the next few months.

Next, I looked at how Samantha uses gestures to communicate. Children usually communicate first with gestures and then add sounds to gestures, which helps them begin to use words. Samantha used only a few clear gestures today. She gave the jar of bubbles and the wind-up toy to you and pushed away the balloon. You reported that she uses only these two gestures at home. Children her age usually also use other gestures, like showing, waving, and pointing. Have you seen her begin to use any new gestures at home? I also noticed that Samantha banged the jar that had Cheerios in it to try to get it open and then got frustrated. It is important for Samantha to learn how to let you know when she needs help, so she won't get frustrated as often. Having more gestures to let you know what she wants will help her right now.

Next, I looked at how Samantha uses sounds. At Samantha's age, children usually use a few different consonants like /m/ and /b/. I didn't hear any consonant sounds used by Samantha today, which is consistent with what you reported at home. She did try to communicate with a grunting vowel sound a few times during the sample, which shows us that she is learning about the importance of the sound as a part of the message. Are there any new sounds she's trying? Is she usually quiet or does she make sounds often?

I also looked at whether Samantha uses words. At Samantha's age, some children will use a few words, but it is not a concern that she is not using words yet. I didn't hear her use any words today, and you reported that she is not yet using words at home. Are there any new words she is trying?

Next, I looked at her understanding of words. Children her age are just beginning to understand a few words. Samantha didn't identify you, point to any body parts, or give me the objects when I named them, but that sometimes happens with very young children. Does she do this at home?

The last thing I looked at was play. I looked at Samantha's play because the way she plays can tell me about what she knows about these objects. Typically, when children begin to use objects functionally, like drinking from a cup or stirring with a spoon, they begin to use their first words. Then, they learn to play with toys toward someone else like a baby doll or stuffed animal as they begin to develop a larger vocabulary. Samantha explored the objects by mouthing them, banging them, and dropping them. This is usually what children do before they begin to use the objects functionally. Children her age usually are using a variety of objects functionally. She was able to stack two blocks, which is very good for her age.

Based on what you reported and what I saw here today, it seems that Samantha is behind in her communication development for her age. She is still very young, so I am encouraged that she will make good progress in the next few months. Although you did not express concern about Samantha's delay in communication development, you may be interested in beginning communication intervention. At Samantha's age, communication intervention would focus on helping her learn how to use eye gaze, facial expression, gestures, and sounds to communicate better, to begin to understand words, and to use objects in play. As she makes gains in these areas, we would then work on her use of words. The next step would be to gather more information in order to decide with you where to begin in intervention. We can provide the intervention in your home, if you would like that, so that the intervention can be built around your daily routines with Samantha. By starting at this young age, Samantha has a better chance to catch up to children her age. We also offer toddler playgroups. They are designed to give you the opportunity to learn how to encourage communication development; you can ask questions, and you will have time to focus on how to play with Samantha."

Guidelines for Reporting the Caregiver Questionnaire and Behavior Sample Results

We have developed a report format for the Caregiver Questionnaire and Behavior Sample. The report includes the child's raw scores, standard scores, and percentile ranks for the composites and total as well as examples of the child's behaviors. For children who perform in the concern range, we recommend reporting "less than the 10th percentile" rather than reporting the specific percentile. An example of the report for Casey is included in Figure 8.6. The organization and wording of these reports should be used as a model for reporting information from the Caregiver Questionnaire and Behavior Sample.

SUMMARY

There is wide variation in the age that children begin talking and the rate that children learn to talk. This makes it difficult to decide when to be concerned if a child is not talking. The sounds and gestures children use to communicate and their ability to understand words and to play with objects provide important clues about their language development. Families are often the first to raise concerns about their child's development. Concerns raised by the majority of families are warranted (Glascoe, 1999); therefore, it is very important to conduct a developmental screening for any child whose family has any concern about his or her development. Some families have concerns about their child even if the child is developing typically. It is important to reassure those families, to provide information about developmental milestones, and to explain their child's development.

Some infants and toddlers are delayed, but families are not yet concerned. It can be difficult for parents to learn that their child is not developing as expected. Due to the degree of inaccuracy of developmental screenings, it is important not to alarm families and to offer support as concerns are raised. It can be confusing to families if one professional tells them that their child is doing fine and another indicates concern; therefore, it is important to coordinate efforts for interdisciplinary evaluations of young children.

The CSBS DP was designed for screening and evaluation of children in the early stages of communication development. Using a parent report tool, such as the CSBS DP Infant-Toddler Checklist, minimizes the time required of health care providers, maximizes the role of the family, and provides reasonably accurate information about whether to refer for a developmental evaluation. The Caregiver Questionnaire and Behavior Sample offer a follow-up evaluation to the Infant-Toddler Checklist and utilize multiple sources of information to build consensus with the family on whether the child has a developmental delay. The parent report tools offer the opportunity to gather information about caregivers' perceptions of what their child can and cannot do as well as concerns about their child. The face-to-face evaluation offers a family-friendly context to evaluate communication skills as well as to observe how the child is functioning in other domains. The CSBS DP offers a clinical tool that supports the use of prelinguistic predictors to improve early identification and maximizes the role of the family in the screening and evaluation process. It should be used with sound clinical judgment to decide whether a child needs further evaluation and/or early intervention and to monitor a child's growth in early communication development.

Child's name: Casey Smith
Date of birth: 5/17/2000
Date of Caregiver Questionnaire: 2/3/2002
Date of Behavior Sample: 2/24/2002
Chronological Age: 20–21 months

Communication Evaluation Report

Casey Smith was referred by his pediatrician for a communication evaluation based on the results of the Communication and Symbolic Behavior Scales Developmental Profile (CSBS DP) Infant-Toddler Checklist, which was completed by his mother, Ms. Barbara Smith. Follow-up information was gathered using the CSBS DP Caregiver Questionnaire and the Behavior Sample.

Findings from the CSBS DP Caregiver Questionnaire

Ms. Smith completed the CSBS DP Caregiver Questionnaire on 2/3/2002. The Caregiver Questionnaire is a 4-page parent report tool used as a follow-up to the Infant-Toddler Checklist, and it asks about the ways that young children communicate before they use words and as they are learning their first words.

The results from this evaluation should be viewed with caution. Although caregivers are likely to be accurate reporters of their children's current and emerging developmental skills, caregivers may over-report or under-report their children's skills. Over-reporting may result in children appearing to have higher skills than what they currently are demonstrating. Under-reporting may result in children appearing to have lower skills than what they currently are demonstrating.

For the following table, a standard score of **6 and below** on a communication skill area or a score of **81 and below** on the total is below what is expected for a child Casey's age. A standard score of 10 and a total score of 100 is considered average.

Communication skill areas	Raw score	Standard score[1,2]	Percentile	
Social Composite	39	8	25	Average
Speech Composite	8	5	<10	Concern
Symbolic Composite	28	7	16	Below average
Total	75	78	<10	Concern

[1] The standard scores are based on a mean of 10 and standard deviation (SD) of 3 for the composite scores and a mean of 100 and SD of 15 for the total score.

[2] Criterion levels for concern are set at more than 1.25 SD below the mean.

Social Composite: This area measures children's abilities to share emotions such as by smiling or frowning, to use eye gaze while interacting, and to use gestures to communicate. It also has questions about why children communicate, for example requesting, showing off, and commenting. Casey smiles, laughs, and looks at adults to express pleasure. His parents are able to tell when he is frustrated or afraid and can comfort him. Casey is using some gestures to communicate, such as pushing an object away, pointing, waving, and shaking his head to indicate "no."

Figure 8.6. Communication evaluation report for Casey.

Speech Composite: This area measures children's use of sounds and words. Casey is using only a limited number of sounds for his age, including /m/, /b/, /d/, and /g/. He is not yet using any words that are understandable to his parents.

Symbolic Composite: This area measures children's understanding of words and their ability to play with objects in ways that are expected for their age. Casey understands at least 19 words, including *mommy, ball,* and *hi*. He is exploring objects and is beginning to play with them doing things like rolling or throwing a ball and pushing a toy vehicle. Casey is not yet pretending with objects or combining actions in play.

Ms. Smith noted that, "Casey was starting to use some basic words several months ago but has not used these words recently." She also noted that, "Casey is very inquisitive and tries to communicate often," but she is concerned that he is not yet using words.

From the information provided on the Caregiver Questionnaire, Casey is communicating below what is expected for his age. Specifically, there are concerns about his use of sounds, words, and play.

Findings from the CSBS DP Behavior Sample

A face-to-face evaluation was conducted with Casey using the CSBS DP Behavior Sample on 2/24/2002. The Behavior Sample provides an opportunity for children to spontaneously communicate with a parent present. The Behavior Sample measures how children communicate before they use words and as they are learning their first words.

The results from this evaluation should be viewed with caution due to Casey's young age. Young children do not always respond optimally when influenced by variables such as unfamiliar settings, hunger, minor discomforts, and shyness. It is common for children's scores to vary across time or from one test administration to the next. The scores provide an estimate of Casey's current developmental skills as seen on the day of the evaluation, but should not be used as predictive measures of his potential.

During the sample, Casey was presented with situations that tempted him to communicate. He was interested but a little sleepy throughout the evaluation session. He frequently displayed shifts in eye gaze between people and objects, and shared emotion by smiling once. Casey used gestures to communicate during the sample. He displayed a high rate of spontaneous communication, which reflects how often he communicated during opportunities presented in the sample.

Ms. Smith reported on the *CSBS DP Behavior Sample: Caregiver Perception Rating Form* that Casey's emotional reaction, attention, comfort level, overall communication, and activity level were typical compared with similar situations. It was reported that Casey's alertness and play behavior were not typical. He was less alert and his play was less organized and focused than usual.

For the following table, a standard score of **6 and below** on a communication skill area or a score of **81 and below** on the total is below what is expected for a child Casey's age. A standard score of 10 and a total score of 100 is considered average.

(Continued)

Figure 8.6. *(continued)*

Communication skill areas	Raw score	Standard score[1,2]	Percentile	
Social Composite	50	11	63	Average
Speech Composite	0	3	<10	Concern
Symbolic Composite	11	3	<10	Concern
Total	61	71	<10	Concern

[1] The standard scores are based on a mean of 10 and SD of 3 for the composite scores and a mean of 100 and SD of 15 for the total score.

[2] Criterion levels for concern are set at more than 1.25 SD below the mean.

Summary of Casey's behaviors observed during the Behavior Sample:

Behavior Sample categories	Examples from Casey's play
Requesting objects and actions	Gave wind-up toy to Mom to wind; reached for the cereal and vocalized "uh" to request the jar; said "uh uh uh" with good inflection to protest his Mom putting a pig in a truck; shook his head "no" to protest the balloon.
Commenting on objects and actions	Pointed to the bird, smiled and said "uh"; waved the Koosh ball and smiled at the clinician to show her the object; tried to pull a frisby out of a toy dog's mouth and said "uh" while looking and smiling at the clnician
Use of a variety of conventional gestures	Giving, showing, pushing away, reaching, pointing, shaking head
Use of a variety of consonants	/n/ and /m/ were noted during the sample, but they were not directed to an adult
Approximations of words	"Mama" was noted but not directed
Comprehension of language	Looked for the pig and pointed to it after Mom encouraged him to put the pig in his truck; showed Mom his toy after the clinician suggested he show her the bird; responded to "Where's Mommy?"; identified two body parts but no objects by name.
Use of organized play behaviors	Put in and stirred; was not very interested in the play set during the sample
Combined play actions	Stirred then put in, one time
Constructive play	Stacked a tower of 5 blocks

Casey demonstrated many early communication skills and emerging language abilities expected for his age. Casey's overall strengths included his ability to:

1. Communicate frequently throughout the behavior sample
2. Direct his mother's attention to objects by showing, waving them, and pointing to them
3. Interact socially by playing Peekaboo
4. Use a variety of gestures

From the information gathered during the Behavior Sample, Casey is communicating below what is expected for his age in sounds, words, and object use. His scores on object use may be underestimating his abilities because of his lack of interest in these play materials.

Conclusions and Recommendations

The information on both the Caregiver Questionnaire and the Behavior Sample indicate that Casey is delayed in aspects of communication development. It is expected that children Casey's age communicate using words. They typically use more than 5 consonant sounds (e.g., /m/, /b/, /p/, /n/, and /t/), use more than 25 different words, and combine words together to make simple phrases (e.g., "more juice," "Mommy open"). By 20 months, children usually imitate words you say, show you body parts, and identify objects when asked. They also will pretend with objects (e.g., feeding a baby doll, cooking with pots and pans). Casey is not yet meeting these developmental expectations. In addition, Ms. Smith reported that "Casey was starting to use some basic words several months ago but has not used these words recently." This is also of concern.

Though some children who are late in talking outgrow this delay, others need early intervention services to help them reach their potential in language and communication abilities (communicate as expected for their age). It is recommended that Casey have a multidisciplinary assessment to determine eligibility for receiving early intervention services offered through Part C of the Individuals with Disabilities Education Act (IDEA) Amendments of 1997 (PL 105-17) and for planning intervention goals and strategies. Based on the information gathered in this evaluation, Casey would benefit from additional support focusing on:

1. Increasing sound and word productions during predictable routines (e.g., using bath time to request and talk about bubbles, boats, water, soap, or duckie).

2. Increasing the variety of actions used with objects in play (e.g., using a spoon to stir, scoop, and feed; using a dump truck to load, carry, and dump).

We will be glad to help you find information sources, reading materials, and professional services that could be beneficial. Please contact our office if you have any questions concerning the information provided or if you need assistance in seeking intervention services. It was a pleasure working with Casey and his family.

Jane Miller, M.S., CCC-SLP
Speech-Language Pathologist

REFERENCES

Angoff, W.H. (1971). Scales, norms, and equivalent scores. In R.L. Thorndike (Ed.), *Educational measurement* (2nd ed.). Washington, DC: American Council on Education.

Bakeman, R., & Gottman, J.M. (1997). *Observing interaction: An introduction to sequential analysis* (2nd ed.). New York: Cambridge University Press.

Baker, L., & Cantwell, D. (1987). A prospective psychiatric follow-up of children with speech/language disorders. *Journal of the American Academy of Child and Adolescent Psychiatry, 26*, 546–553.

Barnett, W., & Escobar, C. (1990). Economic costs and benefits of early intervention. In S.J. Meisels & J.P. Shonkoff (Eds.), *Handbook of early childhood intervention* (pp. 560–582). New York: Cambridge University Press.

Bates, E. (1976). *Language and context: The acquisition of pragmatics.* San Diego: Academic Press.

Bates, E., Bretherton, I., & Snyder, L. (1988). *From first words to grammar: Individual differences and dissociable mechanisms.* New York: Cambridge University Press.

Bates, E., O'Connell, B., & Shore, C. (1987). Language and communication in infancy. In J. Osofsky (Ed.), *Handbook of infant development* (pp. 149–203). New York: John Wiley & Sons.

Bloom, L. (1993). *The transition from infancy to language.* New York: Cambridge University Press.

Bronfenbrenner, U. (1979). *The ecology of human development: Experiments by nature and design.* Cambridge, MA: Harvard University Press.

Brooks-Gunn, J., & Duncan, D. (1997). The effects of poverty on children. *The Future of Children*, 7(2), 55–71.

Bruner, J. (1981). The social context of language acquisition. *Language and Communication, 1*, 155–178.

Carnegie Task Force on Meeting the Needs of Young Children. (1994). *Starting points: Meeting the needs of our youngest children.* New York: Carnegie Corporation of New York.

Coggins, T., & Carpenter, R. (1981). The communicative inventory: A system for observing and coding children's early intentional communication. *Applied Psycholinguistics, 2*, 235–251.

Cohen, J. (1988). *Statistical power analysis for the behavioral sciences* (2nd ed.). Mahwah, NJ: Lawrence Erlbaum Associates.

Crais, E. (1995). Expanding the repertoire of tools and techniques for assessing the communication skills of infants and toddlers. *American Journal of Speech-Language Pathology, 4*, 47–59.

Dale, P., Bates, E., Reznick, J., & Morisset, C. (1989). The validity of a parent report instrument of child language at 20 months. *Journal of Child Language, 16*, 239–249.

Dunst, C., Lowe, L.W., & Bartholomew, P.C. (1990). Contingent social responsiveness, family ecology, and infant communicative competence. *National Student Speech Language Hearing Association Journal, 17*, 39–49.

Education of the Handicapped Act Amendments of 1986, PL 99-457, 20 U.S.C. §§ 1400 *et seq.*

Fenson, L., Dale, P.S., Reznick, J.S., Bates, E., Thal, D., & Pethick, S.J. (1994). Variability in early communicative development. *Monographs of the Society for Research in Child Development, 59*, 1–173.

Fenson, L., Dale, P., Reznick, S., Thal, D., Bates, E., Hartung, J., Pethick, S., & Reilly, J. (1993). *MacArthur Communicative Development Inventories: User's guide and technical manual.* San Diego: Singular Publishing Group.

Florida Starting Points. (1997). *Maximizing Florida's brain power: We need to use it or lose it.* A collaborative project sponsored by the Carnegie Corporation and the United Way of Florida Success by Six.

Glascoe, F.P. (1999). The value of parents' concerns to detect and address developmental and behavioural problems. *Journal of Paediatric Child Health*, 35, 1–8.

Hart, B., & Risley, T. (1992). American parenting of language-learning children: Persisting differences in family–child interactions observed in natural home environments. *Developmental Psychology, 28*, 1096–1105.

Howlin, P., & Rutter, M. (1987). The consequences of language delay for other aspects of development. In W. Yule & M. Rutter (Eds.), *Language development and language disorders.* Philadelphia: Lippincott, Williams & Wilkins.

Hutchinson, T. (1996). What to look for in the technical manual: Twenty questions for users. *Language, Speech and Hearing Services in Schools, 27*, 102–108.

Individuals with Disabilities Education Act (IDEA) Amendments of 1991, PL 102-119, 20 U.S.C. §§ 1400 *et seq.*

Individuals with Disabilities Education Act (IDEA) Amendments of 1997, PL 105-17, 20 U.S.C. §§ 1400 *et seq.*

McCathren, R.B., Warren, S.F., & Yoder, P.J. (1996). Prelinguistic predictors of later language development. In S.F. Warren & J. Reichle (Series Eds.) & K.N. Cole, P.S. Dale, & D.J. Thal (Vol. Eds.), *Communication and language intervention series: Vol. 6. Assessment of communication and language* (pp. 57–75). Baltimore: Paul H. Brookes Publishing Co.

McCathren, R.B., Yoder, P.J., & Warren, S.F. (2000). Testing predictive validity of the Communication Composite of the Communication and Symbolic Behavior Scales. *Journal of Early Intervention, 23,* 36–46.

McWilliam, R.A. & Ware, W.B. (1994). The reliability of observations of young children's engagement: An application of generalizability theory. *Journal of Early Intervention, 18,* 34–47.

Meisels, S. (1996). Charting the continuum of assessment and intervention. In S. Meisels & E. Fenichel (Eds.), *New visions for the developmental assessment of infants and young children* (pp. 27–52). Washington, DC: ZERO TO THREE: National Center for Infants, Toddlers, and Families.

Meisels, S.J., & Wasik, B.A. (1990). Who should be served? Identifying children in need of early intervention. In S. Meisels & J. Shonkoff (Eds.), *Handbook of early childhood intervention* (pp. 605–632). New York: Cambridge University Press.

Messick, S.L. (1989). Validity. In R.L. Linn (Ed.), *Educational measurement* (3rd ed., pp. 13–103). New York: American Council on Education/Macmillan.

Mitchell, S.K. (1979). Interobserver agreement, reliability, and generalizability of data collected in observational studies. *Psychological Bulletin, 86,* 376–390.

Mullen, E. (1995). *The Mullen Scales of Early Learning.* Circle Pines, MN: American Guidance Services.

Mundy, P., Kasari, C., Sigman, M., & Ruskin, E. (1995). Nonverbal communication and early language acquisition in children with Down syndrome and normal development. *Journal of Speech and Hearing Research, 38,* 157–167.

Olswang, L., Rodriguez, B., & Timler, G. (1998). Recommending intervention for toddlers with specific language learning difficulties: We may not have all the answers, but we know a lot. *American Journal of Speech-Language Pathology,* 7, 23–32.

Ounce of Prevention Fund (1996). *Starting Smart: How early experiences affect brain development.* Chicago: Ounce of Prevention Fund.

Paul, R. (1991). Profiles of toddlers with slow expressive language development. *Topics in Language Disorders, 11,* 1–13.

Paul, R., & Jennings, P. (1992). Phonological behavior in toddlers with slow expressive language development. *Journal of Speech and Hearing Research, 35,* 99–107.

Paul, R., Looney, S., & Dahm, P. (1991). Communication and socialization skills at ages 2 and 3 in "late-talking" young children. *Journal of Speech and Hearing Research, 34,* 858–865.

Prizant, B., Audet, L., Burke, G., Hummel, L., Maher, S., & Theadore, G. (1990). Communication disorders and emotional/behavioral disorders in children. *Journal of Speech and Hearing Disorders, 55,* 179–192.

Prizant, B., & Wetherby, A. (1990). Assessing communication of infants and toddlers: Integrating a socioemotional perspective. *ZERO TO THREE, 11,* 1–12.

Rescorla, L. (1989). The language development survey: A screening tool for delayed language in toddlers. *Journal of Speech and Hearing Disorders, 54,* 587–599.

Rescorla, L. (1991). Identifying expressive language delay at age two. *Topics in Language Disorders, 11,* 14–20.

Rescorla, L., & Alley, A. (2001). Validation of the Language Development Survey (LDS): A Parent report tool for identifying language delay in toddlers. *Journal of Speech, Language, and Hearing Research, 44,* 434–445.

Rescorla, L., & Goosens, M. (1992). Symbolic play development in toddlers with expressive specific language impairment. *Journal of Speech and Hearing Research, 35,* 1290–1302.

Rescorla, L., & Schwartz, E. (1990). Outcome of specific expressive language delay (SELD). *Applied Psycholinguistics, 11,* 393–408.

Salvia, J., & Ysseldyke, J.E. (1988). *Assessment in special and remedial education* (4th ed.). Boston: Houghton Mifflin.

Seibert, J., Hogan, A., & Mundy, P. (1982). Assessing social interactional competencies: The Early Social-Communication Scales. *Infant Mental Health Journal, 3,* 244–258.

Squires, J., Potter, L., & Bricker, D. (1999). *The ASQ User's Guide for the Ages & Stages Questionnaires: A parent-completed, child-monitoring system* (2nd ed.). Baltimore: Paul H. Brookes Publishing Co.

Stern, D. (1985). *The interpersonal world of the infant.* New York: Basic Books.

Tabachnick, B., & Fidell, L. (2001). *Using multivariate statistics.* Needham Heights, MA: Allyn & Bacon.

Thal, D., & Tobias, S. (1992). Communicative gestures in children with delayed onset of oral expressive vocabulary. *Journal of Speech and Hearing Research, 35,* 1281–1289.
Thal, D., Tobias, S., & Morrison, D. (1991). Language and gesture in late talkers: A 1-year follow-up. *Journal of Speech and Hearing Research, 34,* 604–612.
Tronick, E. (1989). Emotions and emotional communication in infancy. *American Psychologist, 44,* 112–119.
U.S. Department of Education. (2000). *Twenty-Second Annual Report to Congress on the Implementation of the Individuals with Disabilities Education Act.* (Prepared by the Division of Innovation and Development, Office of Special Education Programs). Washington, DC: U.S. Department of Education.
Walker, D., Greenwood, C.R., Hart, B., & Carta, J. (1994). Prediction of school outcomes based on early language production and socioeconomic factors. *Child Development, 65,* 606–631.
Wetherby, A., Allen, L., Cleary, J., Kwolin, K., & Goldstein, H. (2001). *Validity and reliability of the communication and Symbolic Behavior Scales Development Profile with very young children.* Manuscript submitted for publication.
Wetherby, A., Cain, D., Yonclas, D., & Walker, V. (1988). Analysis of intentional communication of normal children from the prelinguistic to the multi-word stage. *Journal of Speech and Hearing Research, 31,* 24–252.
Wetherby, A., & Prizant, B. (1989). The expression of communicative intent: Assessment issues. *Seminars in Speech and Language, 10,* 77–91.
Wetherby, A. & Prizant, B. (1992). Profiling young children's communicative competence. In S.F. Warren & J. Reichle (Series & Vol. Eds.), *Communication and language intervention series: Vol. 1. Causes and effects in communication and language intervention* (pp. 217–251). Baltimore: Paul H. Brookes Publishing Co.
Wetherby, A., & Prizant, B. (1993). *Communication and Symbolic Behavior Scales, Normed edition.* Baltimore: Paul H. Brookes Publishing Co.
Wetherby, A., & Prizant, B. (1996). Toward earlier identification of communication and language problems in infants and young children. In S.J. Meisels & E. Fenichel (Eds.), *New visions for the developmental assessment of infants and young children* (pp. 289–312). Washington, DC: ZERO TO THREE: National Center for Infants, Toddlers, & Families.
Wetherby, A., & Prizant, B. (1998). *Communication and Symbolic Behavior Scales Developmental Profile, Primary Research Edition.* Baltimore: Paul H. Brookes Publishing Co.
Wetherby, A., Prizant, A., & Barnes, S. (1993). *Communication and Symbolic Behavior Scales Sampling and Scoring Videotapes.* Baltimore: Paul H. Brookes Publishing Co.
Wetherby, A., Prizant, B., & Hutchinson, T. (1998). Communicative, social-affective, and symbolic profiles of young children with autism and pervasive developmental disorder, *American Journal of Speech-Language Pathology, 7,* 79–91.
Wetherby, A., Prizant, B., & Kublin, K. (1995). *Communication and Symbolic Behavior Scales Scoring Tutorial.* Baltimore: Paul H. Brookes Publishing Co.
Wetherby, A., & Prutting, C. (1984). Profiles of communicative and cognitive-social abilities in autistic children. *Journal of Speech and Hearing Research, 27,* 364–377.
Wetherby, A., Yonclas, D., & Bryan, A. (1989). Communicative profiles of handicapped preschool children: Implications for early identification. *Journal of Speech and Hearing Disorders, 54,* 148–158.

A

NORMS TABLES FOR THE CSBS DP INFANT-TODDLER CHECKLIST

INFANT-TODDLER CHECKLIST SOCIAL COMPOSITE SCORES

		n =	50	42	77	126	86	312	296	121	128	174	98	99	133	107	84	87	82	50	36
SS	%ile	Age (months)	6	7	8	9	10	11	12	13	14	15	16	17	18	19	20	21	22	23	24
17	99		17-26	20-26	22-26	25-26	26	26	26	26	26	26	26	26	26	26	26	26	26	26	26
16	98			18-19	21	22-24	23-25	25													
15	95		15-16	15-17	19-20	20-21	22	24	25	25											
14	91		14	14	18	19	20-21	23	24	24	25	25									
13	84		13		17	17-18	19		23	23	24	24	25	25	25	25	25				
12	75		11-12	13	15-16	16	18	21-22	22	22	23		24	24	24	24		25	25	25	25
11	63		10	12	13-14	14-15	17	20	20-21	21	22	23	23	23			24	24	24	24	24
10	50			11	12	13	16	18-19	19	20	21	22	22	22	22-23	23	23	23	23	23	23
9	37		9	10	11	12	15	17	18	19	20	20-21	21	21	21	21-22	22	22	22	22	22
8	25		8	9	9-10	10-11	14	15-16	16-17	17-18	18-19	19	19-20	20	20	20	20-21	20-21	20-21	21	21
7	16			8	8	9	12-13	13-14	14-15	15-16	16-17	18	18	18-19	18-19	18-19	19	19	19	20	20
6	9		7	7	7	8	10-11	10-12	12-13	13-14	15	16-17	16-17	16-17	17	17	17-18	18	18	19	19
5	5		6	6	6	7	8-9	8-9	10-11	11-12	14	14-15	15	15	16	16	16	17	17	17-18	18
4	2		5	5		6	6-7	7	8-9	9-10	9-13	11-13	11-14	13-14	14-15	15	15	15-16	16	16	17
3	1		0-4	0-4	0-5	0-5	0-5	0-6	0-7	0-8	0-8	0-10	0-10	0-12	0-13	0-14	0-14	0-14	0-15	0-15	0-16
SEM 1.1		68% Confidence Interval ± 1.1					90% Confidence Interval ± 1.8					95% Confidence Interval ± 2.1									

INFANT-TODDLER CHECKLIST SPEECH COMPOSITE SCORES

		n =	50	42	77	126	86	312	296	121	128	174	98	99	133	107	84	87	82	50	36
SS	%ile	Age (months)	6	7	8	9	10	11	12	13	14	15	16	17	18	19	20	21	22	23	24
17	99		8-14	8-14	10-14	11-14	12-14	13-14	13-14	13-14	13-14	14	14	14	14	14	14	14	14	14	14
16	98		7		9	10	11	12	12	12											
15	95				8	9	10	11	11	11	12	13	13								
14	91		6	7		8	9	10	10		11	12		13							
13	84			6	7	7				10		11	12		13						
12	75		5				8	9	9		10	10		12	12	13	13	13			
11	63		4	5	6	6				9	9		11	11		12			13	13	13
10	50		3	4	5		7	8	8			9	10	10	11		12	12	12		
9	37			3		5		7	7	8	8		9		10	10-11	11	11	11	12	12
8	25		2		4	4	6	6		7	7	8	8	9	9	9	10	10	10	10-11	11
7	16			2			5	5	6	6		7	7	7-8	8	8	8-9	9	9	9	10
6	9				3	3	4		5	5	6	6	6	6	6-7	7	7	7-8	7-8	8	9
5	5		1	1	2	2		4	4	4	5	5	5	5	5	6	6	6	6	7	8
4	2		0		1		2-3	3	3	3	4	4	4	4	4	4-5	5	5		6	7
3	1			0	0	0-1	0-1	0-2	0-2	0-2	0-3	0-3	0-3	0-3	0-3	0-3	0-4	0-4	0-5	0-5	0-6
SEM 1.0		68% Confidence Interval ± 1.0					90% Confidence Interval ± 1.7					95% Confidence Interval ± 2.0									

INFANT-TODDLER CHECKLIST SYMBOLIC COMPOSITE SCORES

		n =	50	42	77	126	86	312	296	121	128	174	98	99	133	107	84	87	82	50	36
SS	%ile	Age (months)	6	7	8	9	10	11	12	13	14	15	16	17	81	19	20	21	22	23	24
17	99		9-17	9-17	11-17	11-17	14-17	15-17	16-17	16-17	16-17	16-17	17	17	17	17	17	17	17	17	17
16	98		7-8		10	10	12-13	14	15	15											
15	95		6	8	9		11	13	14	14	15										
14	91			7	8	9	10		13			15	16	16	16						
13	84				7	8	9	12	12	13	14	14				16	16				
12	75		5	6	6	7	8	11	11	12	13		15	15	15			16			
11	63			5				10		11	12	13	14	14		15	15		16	16	16
10	50		4	4	5	6	7	9	10	10	11	12			14	14		15	15		
9	37					5		8	9		11	13	13	13		14	14		15	15	
8	25		3	3			6	7	8	9	10	10	12	12	12	13	13	13	14	14	14
7	16				4	4	5	6	7	8	9		11	11	11	11-12	12	12	12-13	13	13
6	9								6	7	7-8	9	9-10	10	10	10	11	11	11	12	12
5	5		2	2	3	3	4	5	5	6	6	6-8	7-8	8-9	8-9	9	9-10	10	10	11	11
4	2		1		2		3	4	4	5	5	5	6	7	7	8	8	8-9	9	9-10	
3	1		0	0-1	0-1	0-2	0-2	0-3	0-3	0-4	0-4	0-4	0-5	0-6	0-6	0-7	0-7	0-7	0-8	0-8	0-10
SEM 1.1		68% Confidence Interval ± 1.1						90% Confidence Interval ± 1.8					95% Confidence Interval ± 2.1								

INFANT-TODDLER CHECKLIST TOTAL SCORES

		n =	50	42	77	126	86	312	296	121	128	174	98	99	133	107	84	87	82	50	36
SS	%ile	Age (months)	6	7	8	9	10	11	12	13	14	15	16	17	18	19	20	21	22	23	24
135	99		33-57	34-57	38-57	45-57	50-57	52-57	52-57	53-57	54-57	55-57	56-57	56-57	57	57	57	57	57	57	57
134	99					44	48-49	51				54	55	55	56						
133	99						47	50	51												
132	98									52	53										
131	98		32						50	51		53				56					
130	98		31	33		40-43	42-46	49	49								56				
129	97			32	37	39	41			50											
128	97							48			52				55						
127	96		26-30			37-38	40	47		49		52									
126	96		25	30-31	36	36			48									56			
125	95			29			39			48	51										
124	95				35				47			54									
123	94		24				38									55	55				
122	93			28	34	35		46		47	50	51		54							
121	92		23	27	33	34		45	46		50	53							56	56	
120	91				32									53	54						
119	90		22			33			45		49	49				54					
118	89				31		37	44					52								56
117	87			26					44	46				52	53			55	55	55	
116	86			25		32		43			48		51			53	54				
115	84						36	42	43												
114	83			24	30	31				45	47	48			52						55
113	81		21				35				46			51				54			
112	79					30		41	42	44			50			52	53		54		
111	77				29	29					45	47		50				53		54	
110	75						34		41	43							52		53		54
109	73			23	28	28	33	40			44	46	49		51					53	
108	70				27				40						51			52			
107	68		20				32	39		42				49					52		
106	66			22				38				45	48		50	50				52	53
105	63			21	26	27		37	39	41	43			48			51				
104	61					26									49			51			
103	58			20	25	25	31	36	38			44	47						51	51	
102	55		19		24					40	42					49	50				52
101	53		18		23	24		35				43			48		49	50	50		51
100	50		17						37	39	41		46	47	47					50	

(continued)

INFANT-TODDLER CHECKLIST TOTAL SCORES *(continued)*

	n =	50	42	77	126	86	312	296	121	128	174	98	99	133	107	84	87	82	50	36
SS	%ile / Age (months)	6	7	8	9	10	11	12	13	14	15	16	17	18	19	20	21	22	23	24
99	47	16		22											48	48				
98	45		19		23	30	34	36	38	40	42	45	46				49			50
97	42													46	47	47		49		
96	40						33	35			41	44	45				48		49	49
95	37				22	29			37	39				45	46					
94	35	15	18			28	32		36		40	43	44			46	47	48	48	48
93	32			21	21			34		38					45			47		
92	30		17								39			44			46	46	47	
91	27			20		27	31	33	35	37		42							46	47
90	25			19				32	34		38		42-43	43		45				
89	23		16			26	30			36		41	41		44	44	45	45		46
88	21	14	15		20		29	31	33			40			43	43	44	44	45	
87	19			18				30		35	37	39	40	42	42	42	43	43	44	45
86	18					25	28	29	32	34							42	42		44
85	16			17	19				31				39	41	41	41			43	
84	14						27	28		33	36	38	38	40	40		41	41		43
83	13			16		24	26		30		35	37		39	39	40	40	40	42	
82	12	13	14		18	23	25		29			36	37	38	38	39				42
81	10				17	22		27	28							38	39	39	41	41
80	9		13			20-21	24			32	34	35	36	37	37	37	38			
79	8			15		19	23	24-26	26-27			34		36			37		40	
78	7			14	16			23	25	31	33		35	35				38		40
77	6					18			24		32	33	33-34		35-36	36	36	37	39	
76	6	12				17	22	22	23	30	31	32	32	34	34	35	35	36	38	39
75	5			13			21							33		34				
74	4	11	12		15			21	22	29		31		32	33	33	34			
73	4		11	12	13-14		20		21		30	30	31		32	32		35		
72	3	10		11	12			20		23-28	29		30	31			33	33-34	36-37	38
71	3		10				18-19		20	22	28	28-29	29	30	31	31	32	32	35	37
70	2	9	9	10		16	17	18-19			27	27	28	28-29	29-30	30				36
69	2	8						17	19	20-21	23-26		27	27	28	29	31			35
68	2						16		18	19	22	23-26			27	28	30	31		
67	1		8	9	10-11						21	22	26	26						
66	1				9	11-15	13-15	16	17	17-18	20		25		26	27	29		33-34	
65	1	0-7	0-7	0-8	0-8	0-10	0-12	0-15	0-16	0-16	0-19	0-21	0-24	0-25	0-25	0-26	0-28	0-30	0-32	0-34

SEM 4.0 | 68% Confidence Interval ± 4.0 | 90% Confidence Interval ± 6.6 | 95% Confidence Interval ± 7.8

NORMS TABLES FOR THE CSBS DP CAREGIVER QUESTIONNAIRE

B

CAREGIVER QUESTIONNAIRE EMOTION AND EYE GAZE CLUSTER SCORES

		n =	12	47	53	71	107	129	114	113	89	55
SS	%ile	Age (months)	6-7	8-9	10-11	12	13-14	15-16	17-18	19-20	21-22	23-24
17	99		14-16	16	16	16	16	16	16	16	16	16
16	98											
15	95			15	15	15	15					
14	91							15	15	15	15	15
13	84			14								
12	75				14	14	14					
11	63		13					14	14	14	14	14
10	50			13	13							
9	37		12			13	13	13	13	13	13	13
8	25		11	12	12							
7	16		10			12	12	12	12	12	12	12
6	9			11	11	11	11					
5	5		9	10	10	10	10	11	11	11	11	11
4	2		8	8-9	9	9	9	9-10	10	10	10	10
3	1		0-7	0-7	0-8	0-8	0-8	0-8	0-9	0-9	0-9	0-9
SEM 0.9		68% Confidence Interval ± 0.9			90% Confidence Interval ± 1.5				95% Confidence Interval ± 1.8			

CAREGIVER QUESTIONNAIRE COMMUNICATION CLUSTER SCORES

		n =	12	47	53	71	107	129	114	113	89	55
SS	%ile	Age (months)	6-7	8-9	10-11	12	13-14	15-16	17-18	19-20	21-22	23-24
17	99		10-20	15-20	18-20	20	20	20	20	20	20	20
16	98			14	17	19						
15	95			13	16		19					
14	91		9	12	15			19				
13	84			11	13-14	18	18		19	19		
12	75		6-8	8-10	12	16-17	17	18	18		19	19
11	63		5	7	11	15	16	17	17	18	18	
10	50		3-4	6	10	12-14	14-15	16	16	17	17	18
9	37		2	5	9	11	13	14-15	15	16	16	16-17
8	25			4		9-10	11-12	13	13-14	15	15	15
7	16			3	7-8	7-8	9-10	11-12	12	13-14	14	
6	9		1	2	6	6	7-8	10	11	11-12	12-13	12-14
5	5				5		6	7-9	7-10	9-10	11	10-11
4	2				4	4-5	5	5-6	6	7-8	8-10	9
3	1		0	0-1	0-3	0-3	0-4	0-4	0-5	0-6	0-7	0-8
SEM 1.0		68% Confidence Interval ± 1.0			90% Confidence Interval ± 1.6				95% Confidence Interval ± 1.9			

CAREGIVER QUESTIONNAIRE GESTURES CLUSTER SCORES

SS	%ile	Age (months) n =	6-7 (n = 12)	8-9 (n = 47)	10-11 (n = 53)	12 (n = 71)	13-14 (n = 107)	15-16 (n = 129)	17-18 (n = 114)	19-20 (n = 113)	21-22 (n = 89)	23-24 (n = 55)
17	99		6-12	10-12	12	12	12	12	12	12	12	12
16	98			9	11							
15	95			8	10							
14	91		5	7								
13	84		4		9							
12	75		3	6	8	10	11					
11	63			5				11	11			
10	50		2	4	7	9	10					
9	37		1	3	6	8				11	11	11
8	25				5	7	9	10	10			
7	16		0	2	3-4	6	7-8	9	9	10	10	
6	9			1	2	5	6	8	8	9	9	10
5	5			0	1	3-4	4-5	4-7	7	8	8	9
4	2				0	1-2	2-3	2-3	3-6	4-7	7	7-8
3	1					0	0-1	0-1	0-2	0-3	0-6	0-6
SEM 1.0		68% Confidence Interval ± 1.0			90% Confidence Interval ± 1.6				95% Confidence Interval ± 1.9			

CAREGIVER QUESTIONNAIRE SOUNDS CLUSTER SCORES

SS	%ile	Age (months) n =	6-7 (n = 12)	8-9 (n = 47)	10-11 (n = 53)	12 (n = 71)	13-14 (n = 107)	15-16 (n = 129)	17-18 (n = 114)	19-20 (n = 113)	21-22 (n = 89)	23-24 (n = 55)
17	99		11-16	14-16	16	16	16	16	16	16	16	16
16	98			13	14-15	15						
15	95			12	13	14	15					
14	91		10	11	12	13	14	15				
13	84		9	10		12	13	14	15			
12	75		8	9	11	11	12	13	14	15	15	
11	63		6-7	8	10	10	11	12	13	14	14	15
10	50		5	7	9		10	11	12	13		14
9	37		4	6	8	9	9		11	12	12-13	12-13
8	25		3	5	7	8		9-10	9-10	11	11	11
7	16		2	4	6	7	7-8	8	8	9-10	9-10	9-10
6	9			3	5	5-6	6	7	7	7-8	7-8	7-8
5	5			2	4	4	5	5-6	5-6	6	6	6
4	2				3	3	4	4	4	5	5	
3	1		0-1	0-1	0-2	0-2	0-3	0-3	0-3	0-4	0-4	0-5
SEM 1.0		68% Confidence Interval ± 1.0			90% Confidence Interval ± 1.6				95% Confidence Interval ± 1.9			

CAREGIVER QUESTIONNAIRE WORDS CLUSTER SCORES

		n =	12	47	53	71	107	129	114	113	89	55
SS	%ile	Age (months)	6-7	8-9	10-11	12	13-14	15-16	17-18	19-20	21-22	23-24
17	99		1-24	8-24	10-24	17-24	17-24	23-24	24	24	24	24
16	98			7	8-9	12-16	16	21-22				
15	95			5-6	7	9-11	13-15	18-20	22-23			
14	91		0	4	5-6	8	12	17	18-21	23		
13	84			3	4	7	10-11	13-16	16-17	22	23	
12	75			2	3	5-6	9	10-12	14-15	20-21	21-22	23
11	63			1	1-2	4	7-8	9	11-13	18-19	18-20	20-22
10	50			0	0	3	5-6	8	10	14-17	15-17	17-19
9	37					2	4	6-7	8-9	11-13	11-14	13-16
8	25					1	2-3	5	5-7	8-10	8-10	10-12
7	16					0	1	4	3-4	6-7	7	8-9
6	9						0	1-3	2	3-5	4-6	4-7
5	5							0	1	2	2-3	3
4	2								0	1	1	2
3	1									0	0	0-1
SEM 1.0		68% Confidence Interval ± 1.0				90% Confidence Interval ± 1.7				95% Confidence Interval ± 2.0		

CAREGIVER QUESTIONNAIRE UNDERSTANDING CLUSTER SCORES

		n =	12	47	53	71	107	129	114	113	89	55
SS	%ile	Age (months)	6-7	8-9	10-11	12	13-14	15-16	17-18	19-20	21-22	23-24
17	99		7-24	15-24	17-24	23-24	24	24	24	24	24	24
16	98			12-14	15-16	21-22						
15	95			10-11	14	19-20	23					
14	91		6	9	13	17-18	20-22	23				
13	84			8	11-12	16	18-19	21-22	23			
12	75		5	7	9-10	12-15	17	19-20	22			
11	63		4	6	8	11	14-16	18	21	23	23	
10	50		3	5	7	9-10	12-13	16-17	19-20	21-22		23
9	37		2	4	5-6	7-8	10-11	14-15	17-18	20	20-22	22
8	25			3	4	6	9	12-13	15-16	17-19	17-19	20-21
7	16		1	2	3	4-5	7-8	10-11	12-14	13-16	13-16	15-19
6	9				2	3	5-6	7-9	8-11	10-12	10-12	12-14
5	5		0	0-1			4	4-6	5-7	7-9	7-9	7-11
4	2					2	3	3	4	5-6	6	6
3	1				0-1	0-1	0-2	0-2	0-3	0-4	0-5	0-5
SEM 1.0		68% Confidence Interval ± 1.0				90% Confidence Interval ± 1.7				95% Confidence Interval ± 2.0		

CAREGIVER QUESTIONNAIRE OBJECT USE CLUSTER SCORES

	n =	12	47	53	71	107	129	114	113	89	55
SS	%ile	Age (months) 6-7	8-9	10-11	12	13-14	15-16	17-18	19-20	21-22	23-24
17	99	5-27	11-27	15-27	22-24	24-27	26-27	27	27	27	27
16	98		9-10	13-14	19-21	23	25	26			
15	95		8	12	18	21-22	24	25			
14	91			11	16-17	20	23	24			
13	84		7	9-10	14-15	18-19	22	23	25-26	26	
12	75	4	6	8	13	15-17	19-21	20-22	24	25	25-26
11	63		5	7	11-12	14	18	19	23	23-24	23-24
10	50	3	4	6	10	13	15-17	17-18	21-22	21-22	22
9	37		3	5	9	11-12	14	16	19-20	19-20	20-21
8	25	2		4	8	9-10	12-13	14-15	16-18	18	18-19
7	16		2		7	8	11	12-13	15	16-17	16-17
6	9			3	5-6	7	9-10	10-11	11-14	14-15	14-15
5	5	1	1	2	4	4-6	6-8	7-9	8-10	11-13	13
4	2				3	3	3-5	3-6	6-7	7-10	10-12
3	1	0	0	0-1	0-2	0-2	0-2	0-2	0-5	0-6	0-9
SEM 1.0		68% Confidence Interval ± 1.0			90% Confidence Interval ± 1.7				95% Confidence Interval ± 2.0		

CAREGIVER QUESTIONNAIRE SOCIAL COMPOSITE SCORES

	n =	12	47	53	71	107	129	114	113	89	55
SS	%ile	Age (months) 6-7	8-9	10-11	12	13-14	15-16	17-18	19-20	21-22	23-24
17	99	30-48	40-48	43-48	46-48	46-48	47-48	48	48	48	48
16	98		38-39	41-42	45	45		47	47	47	
15	95		35-37	39-40	44		46				47
14	91	27-29	32-34	38	43	44	45	46	46	46	46
13	84	25-26	29-31	36-37	41-42	43		45	45		
12	75	22-24	25-28	33-35	39-40	42	43-44	43-44	44	45	45
11	63	21	24	32	37-38	40-41	42	42	43	43-44	43-44
10	50	17-20	22-23	29-31	33-36	37-39	40-41	40-41	42	42	42
9	37	16	20-21	28	32	35-36	38-39	39	40-41	40-41	40-41
8	25		19	27	29-31	33-34	35-37	36-38	38-39	38-39	39
7	16	14-15	16-18	25-26	25-28	28-32	32-34	33-35	36-37	36-37	38
6	9	13	15	20-24	23-24	24-27	30-31	31-32	33-35	34-35	35-37
5	5	11-12	14	18-19	19-22	20-23	21-29	26-30	27-32	30-33	34
4	2	10	13	15-17	15-18	16-19	17-20	18-25	21-26	25-29	27-33
3	1	0-9	0-12	0-14	0-14	0-15	0-16	0-17	0-21	0-24	0-26
SEM 1.0		68% Confidence Interval ± 1.0			90% Confidence Interval ± 1.7				95% Confidence Interval ± 2.0		

CAREGIVER QUESTIONNAIRE SPEECH COMPOSITE SCORES

		n =	12	47	53	71	107	129	114	113	89	55
SS	%ile	Age (months)	6-7	8-9	10-11	12	13-14	15-16	17-18	19-20	21-22	23-24
17	99		11-40	19-40	20-40	31-40	32-40	39-40	40	40	40	40
16	98			17-18	18-19	25-30	30-31	36-38	39			
15	95			14-16	17	22-24	27-29	33-35	37-38			
14	91		10	13	16	18-21	24-26	30-32	32-36	39		
13	84		9	12	14-15	16-17	22-23	26-29	29-31	36-38	38-39	39
12	75		8	10-11	13	15	19-21	22-25	26-28	35	36-37	37-38
11	63		7	9	11-12	14	17-18	20-21	24-25	30-34	32-35	33-36
10	50		6	8	10	12-13	15-16	18-19	22-23	25-29	27-31	30-32
9	37		5	7	9	11	12-14	16-17	18-21	22-24	22-26	25-29
8	25		3-4	6	8	9-10	11	14-15	14-17	18-21	19-21	21-24
7	16		2	4-5	6-7	7-8	10	11-13	12-13	14-17	16-18	16-20
6	9			3	5	5-6	8-9	8-10	9-11	10-13	11-15	12-15
5	5			2	4	4	6-7	6-7	6-8	6-9	7-10	10-11
4	2				3	3	5	5	5	5	6	9
3	1		0-1	0-1	0-2	0-2	0-4	0-4	0-4	0-4	0-5	0-8
SEM 1.1		68% Confidence Interval ± 1.1				90% Confidence Interval ± 1.7				95% Confidence Interval ± 2.1		

CAREGIVER QUESTIONNAIRE SYMBOLIC COMPOSITE SCORES

		n =	12	47	53	71	107	129	114	113	89	55
SS	%ile	Age (months)	6-7	8-9	10-11	12	13-14	15-16	17-18	19-20	21-22	23-24
17	99		12-51	20-51	30-51	41-51	47-51	49-51	50-51	51	51	51
16	98			19	27-29	37-40	45-46	48				
15	95		11	17-18	26	36	39-44	46-47	48-49			
14	91		10	16	21-25	32-35	37-38	44-45	46-47	50	50	
13	84		9	13-15	19-20	28-31	35-36	41-43	44-45	49	49	50
12	75		8	11-12	16-18	24-27	31-34	38-40	41-43	47-48	47-48	49
11	63			10	14-15	21-23	28-30	34-37	39-40	45-46	45-46	46-48
10	50		7	9	13	19-20	25-27	31-33	36-38	41-44	43-44	44-45
9	37		5-6	7-8	11-12	15-18	21-24	27-30	32-35	38-40	40-42	41-43
8	25		4	6	9-10	14	20	24-26	29-31	34-37	34-39	36-40
7	16		3	5	7-8	12-13	16-19	23	25-28	28-33	31-33	34-35
6	9			4	6	11	12-15	18-22	19-24	23-27	23-30	27-33
5	5		0-2	3	5	7-10	10-11	11-17	12-18	15-22	17-22	24-26
4	2			0-2	4	4-6	7-9	8-10	9-11	10-14	13-16	17-23
3	1				0-3	0-3	0-6	0-7	0-8	0-9	0-12	0-16
SEM 1.1		68% Confidence Interval ± 1.1				90% Confidence Interval ± 1.8				95% Confidence Interval ± 2.1		

CAREGIVER QUESTIONNAIRE TOTAL SCORES

SS	%ile	Age (months) 6-7	8-9	10-11	12	13-14	15-16	17-18	19-20	21-22	23-24
	n =	12	47	53	71	107	129	114	113	89	55
135	99	45-139	92-139	112-139	121-139	123-139	131-139	132-139	139	139	139
134	99			107-111		122			138		
133	99			102-106	120	121					
132	98			97-101	117-119	120	130	131			
131	98		72-91	92-96	112-116	119			137	138	138
130	98		71	90-91	107-111	118				137	
129	97			86-89	102-106	117	129	130	136		
128	97		70	82-85	101	116	128				
127	96		69	78-81		115	127		135		
126	96		68	77		114	126			136	
125	95		67	76	100	113	125	129			136-137
124	95		65-66	75		112	124	127-128		135	135
123	94		63-64	74	98-99	111		126	134		
122	93		61-62		97	109-110		125	133	134	
121	92		59-60			108	122-123	124	132		
120	91	44	58		94-96	105-107	121	123	131	133	
119	90			73	91-93	104	115-120	121-122	130		
118	89		55-57		90	103	114	120		132	134
117	87	43	54		87-89	101-102					
116	86				86	100	113	119	129		
115	84		53	72	85	98-99	111-112				133
114	83	42	50-52	71	84	97	109-110	118	128	131	132
113	81		49	70		96	108	117			
112	79	41		69	82-83	95	107	116	127	129-130	130-131
111	77		48	68	80-81		105-106	115	126	128	129
110	75	40			78-79	94	104	112-114	125	127	128
109	73		47	67	77	93		111		126	
108	70	39		65-66	76	90-92	103	110	124	125	127
107	68	38	46	58-64		89	102	109	123	124	
106	66	37		57	75	88	101	108	122	123	126
105	63	36				87	98-100	105-107	121	122	125
104	61	35	45	56	74	85-86	96-97	104	120	121	124
103	58	34	44	55		84	95	103	117-119	119-120	122-123
102	55		43	54	73	83	94		116	117-118	121
101	53		42	53	72	81-82	93	102	115	116	120
100	50	33	41		70-71	80	92				119

(Continued)

CAREGIVER QUESTIONNAIRE TOTAL SCORES

		n =	12	47	53	71	107	129	114	113	89	55
SS	%ile	Age (months)	6-7	8-9	10-11	12	13-14	15-16	17-18	19-20	21-22	23-24
99	47		32	40		68-69	79	91	99-101	111-114	114-115	118
98	45		31	39	52	67		90	98	110	111-113	117
97	42		30	38	51	65-66	78	88-89	97	109	109-110	116
96	40		28-29		49-50	63-64	76-77	86-87	95-96	108	108	115
95	37		27		48	62	75	85	94	106-107	106-107	114
94	35		26	37		60-61	73-74	84		105	105	112-113
93	32		25	36	47	59	72	83	93	103-104	104	110-111
92	30			35			71		91-92	102	103	109
91	27			34	46	58	69-70	81-82	89-90		102	106-108
90	25			32-33		56-57	68	80	88	100-101		104-105
89	23		24	31		55	67	79	87	98-99	101	102-103
88	21			30		54	66	78	85-86	97	98-100	100-101
87	19		23		45	52-53	65		80-84	95-96	97	99
86	18			29	44	51	64	76-77	79	92-94	95-96	98
85	16		22		43	50	62-63	75		91	92-94	96-97
84	14			28	42		61	74	78	87-90	90-91	94-95
83	13			27	41	49	60	73	74-77	83-86	89	93
82	12		21	25-26			59	72	73	82	86-88	88-92
81	10			24	40	48	55-58	71	72	81	84-85	87
80	9			23	39		54		71	80	83	84-86
79	8		20	22	38	47	52-53	67-70	70	79	79-82	82-83
78	7		19	21	37	45-46	51	64-66	66-69	75-78	78	80-81
77	6		18	20	36	43-44	45-50	63	64-65	70-74	77	79
76	6		17		33-35	42	44		63	65-69	69-76	77-78
75	5		16	19	32		43			64	66-68	75-76
74	4		15		31	40-41	42	59-62	62	63	65	74
73	4				30	38-39	41	45-58	58-61	59-62	63-64	73
72	3				29	36-37	40	43-44	50-57	57-58	61-62	72
71	3		14	18	28	33-35	38-39	41-42	42-49	56	59-60	71
70	2				27	31-32	34-37	37-40	41	49-55	55-58	61-70
69	2		0-13		26	29-30	30-33	33-36	40	41-48	50-54	59-60
68	2				21-25	26-28	29	30-32	30-39	33-40	46-49	56-58
67	1			16-17	18-20	22-25	26-28	28-29	28-29	31-32	42-45	53-55
66	1			14-15	16-17	18-21	21-25	22-27	23-27	26-30	38-41	50-52
65	1			0-13	0-15	0-17	0-20	0-21	0-22	0-25	0-37	0-49
SEM 4.0		68% Confidence Interval ± 4.0				90% Confidence Interval ± 6.5				95% Confidence Interval ± 7.7		

C

NORMS TABLES FOR THE CSBS DP BEHAVIOR SAMPLE

BEHAVIOR SAMPLE EMOTION AND EYE GAZE CLUSTER SCORES

		n =	82	76	76	103
SS	%ile	Age (months)	12-14	15-17	18-20	21-24
17	99		18	18	18	18
16	98					
15	95					
14	91		17	17	17	17
13	84					
12	75		16	16	16	
11	63		15	15		16
10	50		13-14	14	14-15	15
9	37		12	13	13	14
8	25		9-11	12	12	
7	16		8	11	11	12-13
6	9		7	9-10	9-10	11
5	5		6	6-8	7-8	10
4	2		4-5	4-5	5-6	8-9
3	1		0-3	0-3	0-4	0-7
SEM 1.0	68% Confidence Interval ± 1.0			90% Confidence Interval ± 1.7		95% Confidence Interval ± 2.0

BEHAVIOR SAMPLE COMMUNICATION CLUSTER SCORES

		n =	82	76	76	103
SS	%ile	Age (months)	12-14	15-17	18-20	21-24
17	99		21-24	22-24	23-24	23-24
16	98		20	21	22	
15	95					
14	91			20	20-21	
13	84		19	19	19	
12	75		18	18		20
11	63		17			19
10	50		16	17	18	
9	37		14-15	16	17	18
8	25		13	14-15	16	17
7	16		10-12	12-13	14-15	16
6	9		6-9	11	13	14-15
5	5		4-5	8-10	8-12	11-13
4	2		2-3	4-7	6-7	10
3	1		0-1	0-3	0-5	0-9
SEM 1.0	68% Confidence Interval ± 1.0			90% Confidence Interval ± 1.7		95% Confidence Interval ± 2.0

BEHAVIOR SAMPLE GESTURES CLUSTER SCORES

		n =	82	76	76	103
SS	%ile	Age (months)	12-14	15-17	18-20	21-24
17	99		19-22	21-22	22	22
16	98		18	19-20	21	21
15	95		17	18	20	20
14	91		16	17	19	19
13	84			16	18	18
12	75		15	15	16-17	17
11	63		14	14	15	16
10	50		12-13	13	14	15
9	37		11	12	12-13	13-14
8	25		9-10	11	11	12
7	16		6-8	8-10	9-10	10-11
6	9		5	7	7-8	7-9
5	5		3-4	5-6	6	6
4	2		1-2	3-4	5	5
3	1		0	0-2	0-4	0-4
SEM 1.0	68% Confidence Interval ± 1.0			90% Confidence Interval ± 1.7		95% Confidence Interval ± 2.0

BEHAVIOR SAMPLE SOUNDS CLUSTER SCORES

		n =	82	76	76	103
SS	%ile	Age (months)	12-14	15-17	18-20	21-24
17	99		20-26	23-26	24	26
16	98		19	21-22	23	
15	95		18	19-20	22	25
14	91		15-17	18	21	24
13	84		13-14	16-17	19-20	23
12	75		12	15	18	21-22
11	63		11	13-14	17	19-20
10	50		7-10	10-12	14-16	17-18
9	37		6	9	12-13	14-16
8	25		4-5	7-8	10-11	10-13
7	16		0-3	4-6	4-9	7-9
6	9			1-3	1-3	4-6
5	5			0	0	1-3
4	2					0
3	1					
SEM 1.1	68% Confidence Interval ± 1.1			90% Confidence Interval ± 1.8		95% Confidence Interval ± 2.1

BEHAVIOR SAMPLE WORDS CLUSTER SCORES

		n =	82	76	76	103
SS	%ile	Age (months)	12-14	15-17	18-20	21-24
17	99		10-28	17-28	27-28	28
16	98		8-9	15-16	25-26	
15	95		6-7	14	23-24	
14	91		4-5	9-13	21-22	27
13	84		3	7-8	16-20	24-26
12	75		2	6	10-15	18-23
11	63		1	5	8-9	15-17
10	50		0	3-4	6-7	11-14
9	37			1-2	4-5	8-10
8	25			0	3	5-7
7	16				1-2	3-4
6	9				0	1-2
5	5					0
4	2					
3	1					
SEM 1.1	68% Confidence Interval ± 1.1			90% Confidence Interval ± 1.8		95% Confidence Interval ± 2.1

BEHAVIOR SAMPLE UNDERSTANDING CLUSTER SCORES

		n =	82	76	76	103
SS	%ile	Age (months)	12-14	15-17	18-20	21-24
17	99		24	24	24	24
16	98		21			
15	95		18			
14	91		15	21		
13	84		9-12	18		
12	75		6	15	21	
11	63			12	18	
10	50		3	9	15	21
9	37			6	12	15-18
8	25		0	3	9	12
7	16			0	3-6	9
6	9				0	6
5	5					3
4	2					
3	1					0
SEM 1.1	68% Confidence Interval ± 1.1			90% Confidence Interval ± 1.8		95% Confidence Interval ± 2.1

BEHAVIOR SAMPLE OBJECT USE CLUSTER SCORES

		n =	82	76	76	103
SS	%ile	Age (months)	12-14	15-17	18-20	21-24
17	99		15-29	20-29	24-29	24-29
16	98			19	23	23
15	95		14	18	22	
14	91		13	17	20-21	21-22
13	84		11-12	15-16	19	20
12	75		10	14	18	19
11	63			13	16-17	17-18
10	50		8-9	12	15	16
9	37		7	11	12-14	15
8	25		6	10	11	13-14
7	16		5	8-9	10	12
6	9		3-4	7	8-9	11
5	5		2	3-6	5-7	9-10
4	2		1	1-2	2-4	7-8
3	1		0	0	0-1	0-6
SEM 1.1	68% Confidence Interval ± 1.1			90% Confidence Interval ± 1.7		95% Confidence Interval ± 2.1

BEHAVIOR SAMPLE SOCIAL COMPOSITE SCORES

		n =	82	76	76	103
SS	%ile	Age (months)	12-14	15-17	18-20	21-24
17	99		55-64	56-64	58-64	61-64
16	98		53-54	55	57	58-60
15	95		52	53-54	56	56-57
14	91		50-51	50-52	54-55	55
13	84		48-49	49	52-53	53-54
12	75		47	48	51	51-52
11	63		44-46	45-47	47-50	49-50
10	50		41-43	42-44	45-46	48
9	37		34-40	40-41	42-44	44-47
8	25		31-33	37-39	38-41	42-43
7	16		27-30	33-36	36-37	40-41
6	9		20-26	31-32	32-35	34-39
5	5		11-19	22-30	22-31	29-33
4	2		9-10	18-21	18-21	26-28
3	1		0-8	0-17	0-17	0-25
SEM 1.1	68% Confidence Interval ± 1.1			90% Confidence Interval ± 1.8		95% Confidence Interval ± 2.1

BEHAVIOR SAMPLE SPEECH COMPOSITE SCORES

		n =	82	76	76	103
SS	%ile	Age (months)	12-14	15-17	18-20	21-24
17	99		28-54	44-54	50-54	54
16	98		27	37-43	46-49	53
15	95		21-26	32-36	44-45	51-52
14	91		18-20	27-31	42-43	48-50
13	84		15-17	23-26	37-41	45-47
12	75		13-14	20-22	29-36	39-44
11	63		11-12	15-19	22-28	33-38
10	50		8-10	13-14	19-21	26-32
9	37		6-7	10-12	16-18	19-25
8	25		1-5	7-9	12-15	13-18
7	16		0	3-6	5-11	8-12
6	9			1-2	4	6-7
5	5			0	1-3	4-5
4	2				0	1-3
3	1					0
SEM 1.1	68% Confidence Interval ± 1.1			90% Confidence Interval ± 1.9		95% Confidence Interval ± 2.2

BEHAVIOR SAMPLE SYMBOLIC COMPOSITE SCORES

		n =	82	76	76	103
SS	%ile	Age (months)	12-14	15-17	18-20	21-24
17	99		35-53	42-53	47-54	48-54
16	98		29-34	40-41	43-46	47
15	95		27-28	38-39	42	46
14	91		23-26	33-37	41	43-45
13	84		19-22	29-32	39-40	42
12	75		15-18	25-28	36-38	39-41
11	63		13-14	22-24	33-35	37-38
10	50		11-12	19-21	26-32	33-36
9	37		9-10	16-18	22-25	30-32
8	25		8	13-15	18-21	26-29
7	16		5-7	11-12	14-17	23-25
6	9		4	7-10	10-13	20-22
5	5		2-3	3-6	5-9	16-19
4	2		1	1-2	1-4	12-15
3	1		0	0	0	0-11
SEM 1.1	68% Confidence Interval ± 1.1			90% Confidence Interval ± 1.9		95% Confidence Interval ± 2.2

BEHAVIOR SAMPLE TOTAL SCORES

		n =	82	76	76	103
SS	%ile	Age (months)	12-14	15-17	18-20	21-24
135	99		113-171	133-171	145-171	150-171
134	99		110-112	132	142-144	149
133	99		109	129-131	141	148
132	98		106-108	127-128		
131	98		103-105	125-126		
130	98		100-102	123-124		
129	97		99	119-122	140	
128	97		98	116-118		147
127	96		97	113-115		
126	96		96	112	138-139	146
125	95		95		137	
124	95		94	111	136	145
123	94		93			144
122	93			110	135	143
121	92		91-92	109		
120	91		90		134	142
119	90			108	133	141
118	89		89			140
117	87		86-88	107	131-132	139
116	86		84-85	103-106	128-130	
115	84		83	101-102	127	138
114	83			99-100	126	137
113	81		81-82	97-98	122-125	134-136
112	79		80	96	121	133
111	77		79	95	119-120	131-132
110	75		78	93-94	118	129-130
109	73		77	91-92	117	128
108	70		76	90	115-116	127
107	68		75	89	113-114	126
106	66		74	88	110-112	124-125
105	63		73		105-109	123
104	61		70-72	87	104	121-122
103	58		69	85-86	102-103	120
102	55		68	84	99-101	
101	53		67	83	97-98	117-119
100	50		66	80-82	95-96	114-116

(Continued)

BEHAVIOR SAMPLE TOTAL SCORES *(continued)*

		n =	82	76	76	103
SS	%ile	Age (months)	12-14	15-17	18-20	21-24
99	47			78-79	94	113
98	45		64-65	77		110-112
97	42		62-63	76	93	108-109
96	40		61	75	92	107
95	37		59-60	74	86-91	104-106
94	35		57-58	72-73	84-85	102-103
93	32		56	69-71	82-83	101
92	30		55	68	81	99-100
91	27		53-54	67	80	97-98
90	25		52	66	76-79	95-96
89	23		51	65	75	93-94
88	21		47-50	64	72-74	91-92
87	19		46	63	71	90
86	18			62	70	86-89
85	16		45	60-61	69	83-85
84	14		42-44	59	67-68	
83	13		41	58	66	82
82	12		40	57	64-65	81
81	10		36-39	55-56	63	79-80
80	9		32-35	54	60-62	78
79	8		31	53	59	77
78	7		29-30	52	56-58	
77	6		27-28	51	55	76
76	6		25-26	50		
75	5		24	48-49	52-54	75
74	4		23	46-47	49-51	
73	4		19-22	43-45	46-48	73-74
72	3		16-18	39-42	43-45	70-72
71	3		13-15	35-38	40-42	60-69
70	2		12	33-34	37-39	51-59
69	2		11	29-32	32-36	49-50
68	2			25-28	27-31	47-48
67	1		10	21-24	22-26	46
66	1		9	17-20	21	45
65	1		0-8	0-16	0-20	0-44
SEM 4.8	68% Confidence Interval ± 4.8			90% Confidence Interval ± 7.9		95% Confidence Interval ± 9.4

BLANK FORMS D

CSBS DP Infant-Toddler Checklist

Child's name: ____________ *Date of birth:* ____________ *Date filled out:* ____________

Was birth premature? ____________ *If yes, how many weeks premature?* ____________

Filled out by: ____________ *Relationship to child:* ____________

Instructions for caregivers: This Checklist is designed to identify different aspects of development in infants and toddlers. Many behaviors that develop before children talk may indicate whether or not a child will have difficulty learning to talk. This Checklist should be completed by a caregiver when the child is between **6 and 24 months of age** to determine whether a referral for an evaluation is needed. The caregiver may be either a parent or another person who nurtures the child daily. Please check all the choices that best describe your child's behavior. If you are not sure, please choose the closest response based on your experience. **Children at your child's age are not necessarily expected to use all the behaviors listed.**

Emotion and Eye Gaze

1.	Do you know when your child is happy and when your child is upset?	❐ Not Yet	❐ Sometimes	❐ Often
2.	When your child plays with toys, does he/she look at you to see if you are watching?	❐ Not Yet	❐ Sometimes	❐ Often
3.	Does your child smile or laugh while looking at you?	❐ Not Yet	❐ Sometimes	❐ Often
4.	When you look at and point to a toy across the room, does your child look at it?	❐ Not Yet	❐ Sometimes	❐ Often

Communication

5.	Does your child let you know that he/she needs help or wants an object out of reach?	❐ Not Yet	❐ Sometimes	❐ Often
6.	When you are not paying attention to your child, does he/she try to get your attention?	❐ Not Yet	❐ Sometimes	❐ Often
7.	Does your child do things just to get you to laugh?	❐ Not Yet	❐ Sometimes	❐ Often
8.	Does your child try to get you to notice interesting objects—just to get you to look at the objects, not to get you to do anything with them?	❐ Not Yet	❐ Sometimes	❐ Often

Gestures

9.	Does your child pick up objects and give them to you?	❐ Not Yet	❐ Sometimes	❐ Often
10.	Does your child show objects to you without giving you the object?	❐ Not Yet	❐ Sometimes	❐ Often
11.	Does your child wave to greet people?	❐ Not Yet	❐ Sometimes	❐ Often
12.	Does your child point to objects?	❐ Not Yet	❐ Sometimes	❐ Often
13.	Does your child nod his/her head to indicate *yes*?	❐ Not Yet	❐ Sometimes	❐ Often

Sounds

14.	Does your child use sounds or words to get attention or help?		❐ Not Yet	❐ Sometimes		❐ Often
15.	Does your child string sounds together, such as *uh oh, mama, gaga, bye bye, bada*?		❐ Not Yet	❐ Sometimes		❐ Often
16.	About how many of the following consonant sounds does your child use: *ma, na, ba, da, ga, wa, la, ya, sa, sha*?	❐ None	❐ 1–2	❐ 3–4	❐ 5–8	❐ over 8

Words

17.	About how many different words does your child use meaningfully that you recognize (such as *baba* for bottle; *gaggie* for doggie)?	❐ None	❐ 1–3	❐ 4–10	❐ 11–30	❐ over 30
18.	Does your child put two words together (for example, *more cookie, bye bye Daddy*)?		❐ Not Yet	❐ Sometimes		❐ Often

Understanding

19.	When you call your child's name, does he/she respond by looking or turning toward you?		❐ Not Yet	❐ Sometimes		❐ Often
20.	About how many different words or phrases does your child understand without gestures? For example, if you say "where's your tummy," "where's Daddy," "give me the ball," or "come here," without showing or pointing, your child will respond appropriately.	❐ None	❐ 1–3	❐ 4–10	❐ 11–30	❐ over 30

Object Use

21.	Does your child show interest in playing with a variety of objects?		❐ Not Yet	❐ Sometimes		❐ Often
22.	About how many of the following objects does your child use appropriately: cup, bottle, bowl, spoon, comb or brush, toothbrush, washcloth, ball, toy vehicle, toy telephone?	❐ None	❐ 1–2	❐ 3–4	❐ 5–8	❐ over 8
23.	About how many blocks (or rings) does your child stack? **Stacks**	❐ None	❐ 2 blocks	❐ 3–4 blocks		❐ 5 or more
24.	Does your child pretend to play with toys (for example, feed a stuffed animal, put a doll to sleep, put an animal figure in a vehicle)?		❐ Not Yet	❐ Sometimes		❐ Often

Do you have any concerns about your child's development? ❐ **yes** ❐ **no** **If yes, please describe on back.**

Communication and Symbolic Behavior Scales Developmental Profile by Amy M. Wetherby & Barry M. Prizant

CSBS DP

CSBS DP Infant-Toddler Checklist: Family Information Form

The following information is needed to contact you for follow-up. This information will remain confidential, meaning that it will not be released to anyone without your written permission.

Child's name: ____________________ *Date filled out:* ____________

Date of birth: ____________ *Age:* ________ *Sex:* ________

Parent's name: ____________________

Address: ____________________

____

Home phone: ____________ *Cell phone:* ____________

Mom's work phone: ____________ *Dad's work phone:* ____________

Describe any complications during pregnancy or your child's birth: ____________

____

____

____

Was your child born premature: ____ *Yes* ____ *No*

If yes, how many weeks early? ____________

Describe any major or recurring health problems your child has had: ____________

____

____

____

____

Describe any concerns you have about your child's development (use back of sheet if needed):

____

____

____

____

INDEX

Page references followed by *f* or *t* indicate figures or tables, respectively.

Communication and Symbolic Behavior Scales Developmental Profile™ Order Form

ORDER THE COMPLETE CSBS DP™ SYSTEM AND SAVE $60!

Includes Test Kit & Toy Kit

Quantity

____ **Complete CSBS DP, First Normed Edition**
Manual, Toy Kit, Forms Package, Sampling Video (VHS), Scoring Video (VHS), and carrying bag
Stock #5494 / Price: $399.00

Quantity

____ **CSBS DP Test Kit, First Normed Edition**—Manual, 25 Infant-Toddler Checklists, 25 Infant-Toddler Checklist: Screening Reports, 25 Caregiver Questionnaires, 25 Caregiver Questionnaire: Scoring Worksheets, 25 Caregiver Perception Ratings, 25 Behavior Sample Worksheets, 1 Outline of Sampling Procedures and Instructions card, 1 Sampling Video, 1 Scoring Video / **Stock #5516 / Price: $199.95**

____ **CSBS DP Toy Kit**—(For owners of CSBS™: All the toys needed to implement CSBS DP are included in the CSBS™ Toy Kit) / **Stock #5524 / Price: $259.95**

TEST KIT ELEMENTS ALSO SOLD SEPARATELY

____ **CSBS DP Manual, First Normed Edition**—**Stock #5567 / Price: $65.00**

____ **CSBS DP Forms, First Normed Edition**—25 Infant-Toddler Checklists, 25 Infant-Toddler Checklist: Screening Reports, 25 Caregiver Questionnaires, 25 Caregiver Questionnaire: Scoring Worksheets, 25 Caregiver Perception Ratings, 25 Behavior Sample Worksheets, and 1 Outline of Sampling Procedures and Instructions card
Stock #5540 / Price: $35.00

____ **CSBS DP Caregiver Questionnaire**—Package of 50 with 50 Scoring Worksheets
Stock #6369 / Price: $25.00 (opened packages of Caregiver Questionnaire are nonreturnable)

____ **CSBS DP Sampling Video**—**Stock #5575 / Price: $50.00**

____ **CSBS DP Scoring Video**—**Stock #5583 / Price: $50.00**

CSBS DP™ Infant-Toddler Checklist and Easy-Score CD-ROM!

This scoring software includes a complete copy of the **Checklist** and comes with a **User's Guide**. Users input responses from the completed **Checklist,** and the program calculates composite percentiles and standard scores based on embedded norms. It also generates a screening report for clinicians to add to the child's health record, and the clinician can select from a menu of three letters to share personalized results and recommendations with the family.

____ **CSBS DP Infant-Toddler Checklist and Easy-Score**—PC-compatible CD-ROM, with User's Guide / **Stock #5605 / Price: $99.95**

❑ Check enclosed (payable to Brookes Publishing Co.)
❑ Purchase Order attached (bill my institution)
❑ Please charge my credit card: ❍ American Express ❍ MasterCard ❍ Visa

Credit Card #: ____________________ Exp. Date: __________
Signature (required with credit card use): ____________________
Name: ____________________ Daytime phone: __________
Street Address: ____________________
Complete street address required. ❑ residential ❑ commercial
City/State/ZIP: ____________________ Country: __________
E-mail Address: ____________________
❑ Yes! I want to receive special web site discount offers! My e-mail address will not be shared with any other party.

Shipping rates for orders within the continental U.S. sent via UPS Ground*
If your product total (before tax) is:

- $0.00 to $49.99, add $5.00
- $50.00 to $399.99, add 10% of product total
- $400.00 and over, add 8% of product total

*For other shipping options and rates, call 1-800-638-3775 (in the U.S. and Canada) and 410-337-9580 (worldwide).

Product Total $________
Shipping Rate (see above) $________
Maryland Orders add 5% sales tax (to product total only) $________
Grand Total U.S. $________

Photocopy this form and mail it to **Brookes Publishing Co.,** P.O. Box 10624, Baltimore, MD 21285-0624, USA; FAX 410-337-8539; call 1-800-638-3775 (8 A.M. – 5 P.M. ET) or 410-337-9580 (outside the U.S. and Canada); or order online at **www.brookespublishing.com**

Policies and prices subject to change without notice. Prices may be higher outside the U.S. Unless otherwise noted, you may return products within 30 days for a full credit of the product price. Refunds will be issued for prepaid orders. Items must be returned in resalable condition.

Your source code is **BA 69**